MADNESS, MALINGERING, and MALFEASANCE

MADNESS,
MALINGERING,
and
MALFEASANCE

**THE TRANSFORMATION OF PSYCHIATRY AND THE LAW
IN THE CIVIL WAR ERA**

R. GREGORY LANDE

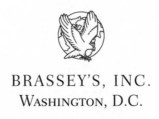

BRASSEY'S, INC.
WASHINGTON, D.C.

Library of Congress Cataloging-in-Publication Data

Lande, R. Gregory.
    Madness, malingering, and malfeasance : the transformation of psychiatry and the law in the Civil War era / R. Gregory Lande.
        p.   cm.
    Includes bibliographical references and index.
    ISBN 1-57488-352-6 (hardcover : alk. paper)
    1. Malingering—United States—History—19th century.   2. Forensic psychiatry—United States—History—19th century.   3. United States—History—Civil War, 1861–1865.   I. Title.
RA1146.L355   2003
614′.1—dc21   2002156574

Printed in the United States of America on acid-free paper that meets the American National Standards Institute Z39-48 Standard.

Brassey's, Inc.
22841 Quicksilver Drive
Dulles, Virginia 20166

First Edition

10   9   8   7   6   5   4   3   2   1

To my family: My mother, Anne, who modeled compassion, my father, Maurice, who taught objectivity, my wife, Brenda, who tirelessly supports our relationship, and the radiant light of my life, my son, Galen.

Contents

ACKNOWLEDGMENTS

N o book ever tells the whole story. Behind the title and beyond the last chapter are many unwritten sentences. These are the invisible contributions that guide, shape, and direct the finished project. Among these is the author's inspiration. Why was this work undertaken? In the case of *Madness, Malingering, and Malfeasance,* the answer is fairly simple: The author has a genuine interest in the historical development of all things medical-legal. The Civil War, America's most costly war, as measured in lives lost, is certainly an important place to begin that study.

The process of bridging the gap between personal interest and scholarly research led the author on a wonderful journey. Along the way, contributors too numerous to mention individually added their own unwritten message to the final work. In some cases these individuals merely pointed the author in the right direction, while others offered much more of their time and advice. A few deserve special recognition for their sustained efforts in promoting the completion of this book. My wife, Brenda, leads the long list of contributors. In addition to providing unflagging encouragement, Brenda repeatedly— and good-naturedly—prepared the manuscript for submission. When my eyes grew bleary reviewing the manuscript, a second set of eyes—Brenda's—took over. Her expertise as a librarian was an indispensable asset when I was doing the research for this book. My son, Galen, deserves credit, too. Evidencing a maturity exceeding his teenage years, he proved to be an insightful critic.

There were many trips to the National Archives, various libraries, and rare book dealers. Each one contributed a piece, which, taken together, completed a picture of medical jurisprudence, as it existed during America's Civil War.

Of course no work makes the transition from author's desk to publication without a publisher's commitment. This entails a calculated assessment by the publisher in deciding which of many meritorious submissions to support. Brassey's extended such confidence to this project. The editorial staff, in the person of David Arthur, then provided the professional coaching that fine-tuned this book.

As a result of these combined efforts, the historical evolution of the unique professional collaboration between medicine and the law, as it existed during the Civil War, can be seen as an important foundation on which modern concepts of medical jurisprudence were built.

PREFACE

Genealogy is a popular pursuit that establishes historical lineage. From some distant union, the researcher seeks an unbroken line from the past to the present. The history of forensic psychiatry can be traced in a similar fashion. The birth of this profession is the consequence of a practical relationship between medicine and the law. As both professions matured, there were times when interests overlapped, resulting in brief cooperative mergers. These early embraces nurtured the embryonic growth of forensic psychiatry.

Unearthing the roots of forensic psychiatry required considerable digging. Historically, medicine and the law have pursued separate paths, but as medicine began to study human behavior, previously inexplicable criminal acts came to be defined in rudimentary scientific terms. An insane individual, for example, might steal seemingly useless items as the result of a mental illness that robbed him of his rational faculties.

Modern criminal courts are still bewildered in their attempts to distinguish the boundaries among madness, malingering, and malfeasance. Experts in human behavior now routinely assist the judicial system in distinguishing these boundaries, and the outcome of these deliberations often determines a defendant's fate.

Identifying and selecting material for this book was dependent on the discovery of examples of madness, malingering, and malfeasance that resulted in a military prosecution. This was a rather painstaking process that required many hours sifting through documents at the National Archives and through special library collections at the Pentagon, the Library of Congress, and the National Library of Medicine. Certain sections of the National Archives, such as Record Group 48, offered a relative treasure trove of relevant material. The admission logs for the Government Hospital for the Insane, stored in Record Group 418, held clues about individuals who had been committed for mental treatment following some form of criminal conduct. Official military records of the Civil War era, including government orders and court-martial proceedings, were selected for study when the case involved insanity or a question of criminal competency.

Only a few scattered references to prosecuted malingering were uncovered.

Malfeasance, on the other hand, was amply documented during the Civil War Era. The stories chosen for inclusion in *Madness, Malingering, and Malfeasance* were those where mental illness or severe alcohol abuse were present and contributed to misconduct. Military courts responded to similar cases unequally, although glimpses of the future cooperation between medicine and the law can be seen in some court-martial proceedings.

The intent of *Madness, Malingering, and Malfeasance* was not to catalog every example of these behaviors and their associated legal outcomes, but instead to present sufficient information portraying the embryonic origins of forensic psychiatry. The Civil War Era parents of forensic psychiatry—medicine and the law—would barely recognize the modern fruits of their union.

INTRODUCTION

D uring the Civil War the sounds of battle masked a different struggle. Exploding ordnance, anguished cries, and desperate commands drowned out the quieter conflict of emotional disorder. Although those with national political motivations recognized the competing conflict, they accepted the need to muffle it, believing that silence somehow could inhibit the contagion. While combat directly engages the opponent, the other struggle fought during the Civil War was against an intangible enemy. Losses on the battlefield are measured with certainty, but the intangible enemy strikes armies from within. If left unchecked, emotional problems can cause personnel losses to multiply, gaps in military readiness to widen, and critical battles to be lost before they are fought.

Military leaders understood the threat, but traditional weapons were useless against it. The debilitating killer, acting through madness, malingering, and malfeasance, effectively neutralized many combatants. The men who suffered severe emotional problems were lost to hospitals, many more committed crimes like desertion, while others simply invented an illness for themselves, the combination resulting in a progressive shortfall of soldiers. Further losses were

1

incurred when precious other human resources were diverted to control the consequences of madness, malingering, and malfeasance. Instead of fighting, for example, some soldiers were in perpetual pursuit of their absent comrades.

A national campaign strategy was essential. Military commanders, lawyers, and physicians joined with civilian leaders in creating a loosely linked program to stem these losses. Components of the program included military laws, effective leadership, punishment, and medical treatment.

The cooperative alliance among the military, medical, and legal professions, perhaps not formally recognized as such, existed functionally to prevent losses from these causes. Military commanders contributed through leadership; successful leadership inspired confidence, enhanced morale, and provided purpose to combat. Using control, executed through military orders, a commander maintained discipline and obedience. By understanding his men, a good leader was able to strike a careful balance between obedience and incentive, which in turn earned the commander the respect of his men. The harshness of military life was tempered by this reciprocal respect and surely contributed to the cohesive group spirit that is necessary to wage war.

Prudent military commanders engaged civilian authorities—war rarely recognizes boundaries that shield civilians. Those left at home not only faced an uncertain fate, they were also expected to bear the brunt of equipment and supply shortages that were taken to support the military. Mobilizing civilian patriotism helped insulate the populace from many hardships. A military-civilian compact was essential to maintaining combat readiness, which was particularly important during the Civil War.

Induction, retention, and social control were three pivotal areas that required cooperation. Civilian collaboration was essential to attract, and later draft, military personnel. Retention focused civilian efforts on preventing and retrieving personnel losses resulting from unauthorized absences from military duty. Social control enlisted the citizenry in a moral crusade, the goal of which was to immunize the troops against certain vices such as alcohol, gambling, and prostitution.

A legal system was in place to reinforce a military commander's personal leadership style. The military legal system shaped behavior that promoted the commander's goal of prosecuting a war. Military attorneys, referred to as judge advocates, not only prosecuted crimes, they also provided expert legal advice to commanders. The accused—a military person charged with a crime—was granted specific limited safeguards that served to protect against prosecutorial bias. Expedience, forced by war, tested the impartial resolve of the military legal system during the Civil War.

Fielding an army and defeating the enemy required bullets, not laws, or so some leaders seemed to believe. This shortsighted approach trivialized one of the most important aspects of military law, that of legitimizing the exercise of authority. There should be no shortcuts on the path to justice, although many were taken during the Civil War. Too often leaders traded political advantage or expedience for fairness. The number of executions, for example, peaked as politicians sought in vain to stem the instances of desertion. Soldiers stood before the bar of justice without legal counsel, and many mentally ill defendants were punished, not treated. Fortunately, the medical and legal communities learned lessons from these unfortunate circumstances and progressively adopted procedures to prevent their reoccurrence.

The gradual professionalization of the military medical-legal system is recorded in soldiers' letters and diaries, various government publications, courts-martial transcripts, and hospital documents. A study of the professional practices that were prevalent before the Civil War and the lessons that were learned as a result of the conflict demonstrates a steady growth and maturation of the system. From this study, an uneven, but progressive, trend favoring compassion and justice emerges.

The influence of civilian medical jurisprudence was definitely on the wane in the quarter century before the Civil War began.[1] Several factors contributed to the malaise, not the least of which was economic in origin—physicians resented spending time in trials without receiving a reasonable remuneration. Also, a number of sensational cases generated great controversy, hindering the advance of medical jurisprudence. One of the most famous involved an English defendant by the name of Daniel McNaughton, who was at the center of a celebrated insanity trial in 1843.[2] The lessons learned from this criminal trial were so important that the principles crossed boundaries and oceans, with America and her military both absorbing the lessons. Insanity cases were rarely brought to court, but when they were, any subsequent such case would come across the name of Daniel McNaughton.

The McNaughton trial was the subject of daily newspaper coverage, which was uniformly unsympathetic. McNaughton reportedly had an unusual childhood history, and newspaper reports speculated that a strained father–son relationship had warped his later behavior. Although the fact that McNaughton was born out of wedlock remained a dark family secret that was rarely discussed, various behavioral clues began to emerge. There were, for example, over a period of many years, innumerable instances when favors bestowed upon the other children were pointedly denied him. These perpetual minor insults paved the way for the ultimate rebuke—McNaughton's father refused his son a stake in the family business, essentially ejecting him from the family and forcing him to learn a trade.

Shortly after leaving home, McNaughton began experiencing severe headaches, which were accompanied by a developing sense of persecution. All his life McNaughton had suffered: Through no fault of his own, he had been shunned and ridiculed, and now he was tortured by headaches. A mind made vulnerable by constitution and molded by life circumstances gradually warped. It was reported that McNaughton increasingly blamed his distress on the police or the church, claiming he was the object of their persecution. Initially, these thoughts of persecution were loosely organized. McNaughton traveled to France, apparently in an attempt to hide from his tormentors; however, no relief attended the move. Instead, it was his belief that the conspiracy followed him.

McNaughton returned to England, seemingly convinced that unseen agents were seeking his downfall. He complained to the local constabulary, but, far from gaining confirmation or protection, McNaughton was branded insane. His family was informed, and characteristically, they ignored his predicament.

The loosely organized paranoia eventually coalesced and took a threatening turn. McNaughton came to believe that he was a target because he had voted against the ruling party in the preceding political election. His disordered mind reasoned that the ruling party's vengeance was at the source of his suffering. His feverish mind conjured all sorts of perils, resulting in McNaughton's firm belief that his life was in danger and he had no alternative but to defend himself.

McNaughton moved to London, with the apparent goal of killing Sir Robert Peel, an important person, respected as the founder of a modern police force and as a member of the ruling party. McNaughton's plan would have been flawlessly executed, except for the fact that he missed his intended target and shot the wrong person. The London newspaper headlines screamed their outrage. Edward Drummond, Sir Robert Peel's secretary, had been wantonly murdered on January 20, 1843.

Ostensibly, McNaughton incriminated himself shortly after his arrest, when he firmly accused the ruling party. "They follow and persecute me wherever I go, and have entirely destroyed my peace of mind. . . .They have accused me of crimes of which I am not guilty; in fact they wish to murder me."[3]

Daniel McNaughton sought refuge from the murder charge by claiming insanity. A distinguished barrister by the name of Alexander Cockburn, who was familiar with a handful of English insanity cases, represented him. A favorable verdict for the defense was rare in British courts, which generally excused only the most severely disturbed defendants—those indistinguishable mentally from "a wild beast."[4]

It was the prosecution's position that McNaughton was not severely impaired, and they dwelled extensively on his deliberation, planning, and public comments. Witnesses testified that McNaughton pursued rational interests, such as studying complex academics and operating a business. The prosecution firmly contended that, although McNaughton could be moody and withdrawn, those characteristics hardly disturbed his daily activities.

Further condemning the defendant were eyewitness accounts placing him near the residence of Sir Robert Peel for a period of two weeks before the crime was committed. When questioned about these reports, he invariably invented plausible lies.

The prosecution was confident. There were no distinguishing characteristics to separate McNaughton's acts from those of a sane person, and the prosecution was of the opinion that there was no need to call medical experts to explain the obvious. That decision turned out to be a mistake.

Adopting a legal strategy designed to advance a more liberal definition of insanity, McNaughton's attorney probed his client's behavior. Citing an eminent text of criminal evidence, Cockburn sought to prove that, "a mad person may be perfectly aware that murder is a crime, and will admit it, if pressed on the subject; still he may conceive that the homicide he has committed was nowise blamable, because the deceased had engaged in a conspiracy, with others, against his own life, or was his mortal enemy, who had wounded him in his dearest interests, or was the devil incarnate, whom it was the duty of every good Christian to meet with weapons of carnal warfare."[5]

Cockburn assembled an impressive group of witnesses: McNaughton's family generously illustrated his complicated childhood; the sheriff remembered McNaughton's raving behavior at the time of his arrest; four medical witnesses testified as to his mental state—two of the doctors personally examined McNaughton, and the other two testified solely on the basis of courtroom observations. Their collective testimony was important.

Cockburn's study of McNaughton's life exposed a deeply troubled soul, with the most pronounced changes occurring as McNaughton approached manhood. Reportedly, he became withdrawn and irrational, a change in his personality that mystified his family. In a moment of confidence, his father first learned that McNaughton believed he was being "followed." His father listened incredulously as his son fearfully described the spies. Acting on this belief, McNaughton took steps to elude his persecutors. He took a brief trip to France to escape his tormentors, but found he was unsuccessful when he "saw" them awaiting him at the boat dock. McNaughton fled back to Britain, and his mental deterioration continued its downward spiral. Just before the murder of Drummond, McNaughton was forced from his lodgings, because his fellow lodgers had been both alarmed and annoyed by his strange utterances and nocturnal screams.

Dr. E. T. Monro had carefully evaluated McNaughton at the request of McNaughton's defense counsel. There was no doubt from his testimony what he thought:

> The prisoner said he was persecuted by a system . . . [and] wherever he went; that he had no peace of mind, and he was sure it would kill him; that it was grinding of the mind. I asked him if he had availed himself of medical advice? He replied, that physicians could be of no service to him . . . he observed people in the streets pointing at him, and speaking of him . . . everything was done to associate his name with the direst of crimes . . . he was perpetually watched and followed. . . . His complaints had been sneered and scould [sic] at by Sheriff Bell, who had it in his power to put a stop to the persecution . . . he was afraid of going out after dark, for fear of assassination . . . he had seen paragraphs in the *Times* newspaper containing allusions which he was satisfied were directed at him . . . he had seen articles . . . insinuating things untrue and insufferable of him; that on one or two occasions something pernicious had been put into his food.[6]

Clearly, McNaughton was suffering from a delusion—an immutable belief that controlled his behavior. Although the belief was irrational, it nevertheless forced the victim's compliance; in essence, McNaughton was enslaved by this mental duress. As a consequence, McNaughton reasoned that his life was at risk and he acted in self-defense. The two physicians who carefully followed the trial, observing McNaughton throughout, were convinced that he was delusional.

The evidence phase of McNaughton's trial came to an end, and all that remained was the determination of a verdict. After receiving the judge's instructions, the jury deliberated rather briefly before announcing McNaughton was "not guilty, on the grounds of insanity."

The nation had followed the case closely, and the verdict unleashed a firestorm of public protest. Newspapers fanned the flames by publishing incendiary rebukes. "Ye people of England exult and be glad, for ye're now at the will of the merciless mad."[7]

Queen Victoria added her comments to the public voice of discontent, when she criticized the English legal system for allowing this immoral verdict. The Queen's criticism spurred a legislative review of the insanity defense, whereby fifteen judges were impaneled to critique, and recommend changes to, the insanity defense. After deliberation, the justices presented their version of a model insanity defense: "To establish a defense on the ground of insanity, it must be clearly proved that, at the time of the committing of the act, the party accused was laboring under such a defect of reason, from disease of the mind, as not to know the nature or quality of the act he was doing; or if he did know it, that he did not know that he was doing what was wrong."[8] The proposed insanity defense eventually became known as the McNaughton standard.

Fewer than twenty years after Daniel McNaughton's case rocked Great Britain, the United States experienced a similar controversy in 1859. New legal ground was broken when Daniel Sickles introduced the nation to the idea of temporary insanity.[9]

Daniel Sickles was a powerful New York Congressman, whose sphere of influence apparently did not extend to his wife, who preferred the company of Philip Key, the son of Francis Scott Key, over that of the Congressman.

Sickles accosted Key in broad daylight, on a public thoroughfare, across the street from the White House. Heated words were exchanged between the two, and Sickles drew a firearm, wounded Key, and then, as his victim lay helpless on the ground, Sickles killed him. Following the murder, Sickles calmly turned himself in to the local police.

Edwin M. Stanton, the future Secretary of War for President Abraham Lincoln, conducted Sickles's defense. Without a blush, Stanton spent the next month portraying his client as having been temporarily insane when the murder was committed. Stanton's definition of insanity conveniently excluded mental illness. Instead, passions stoked by jealousy and anger were offered as evidence of an "illness" that robbed Sickles of his judgment. Stanton brilliantly positioned his client as the victim of infidelity and offered no medical testimony. After several weeks, the trial finally concluded, and the jury deliberated for only a few minutes. Sickles was found not guilty.

The national obsession that accompanied Sickles's trial soon gave way to a sober reflection. The definition of insanity had been stretched to the point where the perpetrator of any premeditated crime—in the hands of a skillful attorney—could be exonerated of misconduct. Public confidence in medical jurisprudence plummeted and was not revived until the Civil War.

Just prior to the Civil War, medical jurisprudence—the reciprocal investment between the medical and legal professions—was nonexistent. Both were in a state of sleepy repose, given the small size of the military force. Nonetheless the military legal system seemed poised to take advantage of medical contributions. Military training and tradition had favored the team approach to problem resolution since America's birth.

During the period of fewer than one hundred years between Colonial times and the beginning of the Civil War, notable changes occurred in military law. By 1775, years of simmering resentment had reached the boiling point, and the thirteen British colonies in America demanded independence. The fledgling Continental Congress understood that a simple declaration of independence was, by itself, insufficient. Wresting independence from Great Britain would require force, which could only be exerted through the creation of a Continental Army. Preliminary steps were taken that year, and the Second Continental Congress approved a military code in 1775.[10] There were sixty-nine articles in America's first military code, which were created by blending elements of British tradition with the previously existing Massachusetts Articles of War. These sixty-nine articles provided a general framework for conducting all aspects of military operations.

The Military Code of 1775 was reorganized one year later.[11] The specter of war that was haunting the colonies had unmasked a curious omission in the original military code—the mention of anything to do with espionage. War heightens vigilance and encourages clandestine activities. Through the use of spies, enemy nations hope to pry secrets loose, and the resulting damage can be immense. Spies have the capacity to burrow deep into and collapse an operation. The Military Code of 1776 rectified the omission and condemned spies, calling for convicted spies to face the death penalty.

The Military Code was a living document that matured with America. In the decade following the birth of the United States, for the most part, only minor amendments were made to the Code. A major growth spurt occurred in the development of the military law in 1786.[12] Although the first war with Great Britain was over, tensions remained, but eventually subsided to a level that permitted some reduction in the number of American forces. The Military Code of 1786 addressed the needs of smaller units; in particular, the quorum necessary to dispense justice was altered. It was decided that courts-martial in smaller units could be conducted with fewer members than had previously been done. That decision considerably eased the burden of assembling and monopolizing the time of limited numbers of personnel.

The Military Code was again amended in 1806, adopting one hundred and one articles, along with extra punishment for spies.[13] This was an enduring revision that lasted through the Civil War. In its thirty-one years of life, the Military Code had grown from sixty-nine to one hundred one articles.

In addition, there were several authoritative texts on military law. The authors of these works interpreted, clarified, and expanded the simple Articles of War, which constitutionally administered military demeanor. Titles such as *Benét's Treatise on Military Law*, *O'Brien's Treatise on American Military Law*, and later, the influential *Win-*

throp's *Military Law and Precedents* were available to lawyers. These books introduced the novice to the basics of military law, and that practical introduction was followed by a comprehensive analysis. A vast array of regulations, government orders, and courts-martial added to the body of information on military law. All of these sources were valuable in organizing a legal defense.

Two types of courts-martial were recognized by military law—general and garrison, or regimental—which differed in quorum and legal jurisdiction. The preferred military trial was a general court-martial, which was created solely through the service of commissioned officers. Thirteen officers sat in judgment, except during times where assembling that number would negatively affect military readiness. In such instances, the Articles of War allowed as few as five officers to constitute a general court-martial. A general court-martial enjoyed full jurisdiction and was empowered to try any crime and invoke capital punishment.

The garrison, or regimental, court-martial was more limited in scope. It was convened with only three officers, who could neither try capital cases nor prosecute a fellow officer. Soldiers convicted by a garrison, or regimental, court-martial could not receive a fine exceeding one month's pay or be confined for longer than one month.

The judge advocate, who generally represented the government, was forced to straddle a hopeless conflict of interest. His chief responsibility was to prosecute; however, under military law, he was also charged with the competing responsibility of serving as counsel for the defense. The prosecutor "shall so far consider himself as counsel for the prisoner, after the said prisoner shall have made his plea, as to object to any leading question to any of the witnesses, or any question to the prisoner, the answer to which might tend to criminate himself."[14] The military did not provide a dedicated defense counsel for the accused, however, a soldier could hire a private defense attorney, if he had the means.

Several articles regulated punishment.[15] Courts-martial were prohibited from sentencing an offender to more than fifty lashes. Officers convicted of cowardice, and subsequently cashiered, suffered additional humiliation: Article 85 required that the crime be publicized "in the newspapers in and about the camp, and of the particular state from which the offender came."

Each officer serving on a court-martial was made to swear an oath administered by the judge advocate, requiring members to judge the accused only according to the evidence and the law. Members were admonished to banish favoritism from their deliberations.

Courts-martial unfolded in a manner recognizable to any civilian attorney. The jury members, president, and judge advocate were all selected in advance of the actual trial. On the first day of trial, the convening order authorizing the court-martial was duly recorded. With all participants in the court, this might have been the first opportunity for the accused to survey his jury. Article 71 allowed the accused to challenge a court member, after which the court would briefly consider the reasons given for the challenge and make its determination.[16] Following this rarely invoked legal right, the judge advocate would read the charges and specifications, the prisoner would enter a plea, and, barring any further complications, the trial would begin.

Unless military conditions dictated otherwise, trials were conducted "between the hours of eight in the morning and three in the afternoon." All members and observers were admonished to maintain a calm decorum, or face punishment for the disturbing conduct.[17]

The prosecution presented its witnesses first, and they were sworn in with the following statement. "You swear, . . . the evidence you shall give in the cause now in hearing shall be the truth, the whole truth, and nothing but the truth. So help you God."[18] Following the pledge, the judge advocate, court members, accused, and, lastly, his attorney, in turn questioned each prosecution witness. In a similar pattern, the defense would then present its witnesses. After the defense rested their presentation, the accused was entitled to make a statement to the court members.

A verdict was presented only after the court members swore an oath ensuring that evidence was examined, "without partiality, favor, affection, prejudice, or hope of reward."[19] Noncapital cases required a simple majority for conviction, but Article 87 set the bar higher for the death penalty.[20] For the ultimate punishment, two-thirds of the members had to agree.

Opportunities to appeal a verdict were limited. The commanding officer that convened the court-martial could either pardon or mitigate a sentence. A death sentence could be pardoned or mitigated by the appropriate convening officer, or "in the case where he has the authority to carry them into execution, he may suspend, until the pleasure of the President of the United States can be Known."[21] A verbatim record of the court-martial accompanied appeals for clemency.

Similarities between civilian and military trials offered most attorneys a measure of comfort. The procedure was familiar and required no great change in practice. There were peculiarities of course, such as court members examining witnesses. Many of the crimes had no counterpart in civilian courts, yet, those offenses were clearly tied to the imperative to maintain control. On the whole, the process afforded a fair structure to present a defense.

Military laws, regulations, and court opinions collectively suggested strategies for planning the best defense.[22] Legal defenses recognized by military law were broadly grouped into two classes. The first strategy to rebut an accusation attacked the prosecution's evidence. Fortunately, even the same set of facts could hold different interpretations, emphasizing just how complex behavior is. A smart attorney, for example, could introduce reasonable doubt by first accepting the basic evidence. By reassembling that evidence the defense attorney could give jury members a different story built on the same set of facts. An accused deserter, for example, might admit his unauthorized absence. The crime of desertion required that the prosecution prove the soldier harbored a permanent intent to leave the military. More than one defendant accused of desertion attacked the intent issue by solemnly declaring that their absence had been temporary. If the accused was gone for a longer period, he could always insist he was lost, on a secret mission, duped by a confederate, or perhaps responding to an urgent letter from home. The success of the accused to get charges dropped often revolved around the believability of his explanation, although a dash of contrition was also helpful.

Another way to introduce doubt was to remove the accused from the scene of the misconduct, that is, establishing an alibi for him by providing eyewitness testimony that placed him somewhere other than the scene of the crime. Such testimony could undermine a key part of the prosecution.

The second broad category of defense strategies tackled the legal definition of a crime. Experienced criminal attorneys understood that two ingredients were required to label misconduct as criminal. First, the prosecution had to prove that the defendant had committed an illegal act, the *actus reas*, in legal parlance. The prosecutor bore the additional responsibility of proving the defendant had committed the foul deed under sway of an evil mind, *mens rea,* as it was legally known. Accidental acts, even if they caused considerable harm, were done without wicked intent and were not considered crimes. The formula for criminal prosecution, then, required an illegal act to have been committed with evil intent.

Many defense strategies aim to mitigate criminal intent. Perhaps the least successful argument, or at least most skeptically received, claims ignorance. The military endorsed the presumption that ignorance of a particular law was no excuse for misbehavior. Officers in particular were schooled in military rules, all but obviating reliance on such a criminal defense; however, enlisted soldiers, many who could not read or write, might at least entertain the option. Article 101 minimized any optimism hoped for from the use of this tactic by requiring that the military code "be read and published once in every six months to every garrison, regiment, troop or company in the service of the United States."[23] A faithful unit's allegiance to this directive would hardly support a claim of ignorance. Military courts-martial were familiar with this tactic and were rarely sympathetic. Even foreign soldiers who donned the U.S. uniform and spoke English poorly found little relief by claiming ignorance of the law.

The actual practice of military law often fell short of adhering to the written code. Fortunately, the military medical and legal professions both moved forward and became more refined. Just as Napoleonic tactics and antiquated weaponry gave way to advances in military science, so were similar changes made in the practice of medical jurisprudence. Early controversies regarding medical care, the role of alcohol, treatment of the mentally ill soldier, prosecution of crime, and methods of punishment all eventually yielded to innovative thinking during the years America bled and died, and the gains continued after the war ended. America had discovered that compassion and justice could coexist with a national emergency. Ultimately, all wars are won at home. The nation that battles injustice destroys an enemy that can surely sabotage all other efforts.

CHAPTER ONE

———◆———

U.S. v. STEWART

In 1863 Pvt. Leroy Shear joined the 14th Artillery Regiment in Rochester, New York.[1] Dissatisfied with the unit, he deserted it after a month, traveled to Utica, and became a substitute. To cover his trail, Private Shear adopted an alias to conceal his true name. His nom de guerre stuck, and all future reports adopted his new name, Lorenzo Stewart. Despite his desertion, Stewart maintained an interest in military service. Casting off his given name along with his old unit, Stewart enlisted as a substitute in the place of one Jacob Smith.[2] Smith never inquired, and Stewart never divulged, that he had not been discharged from his first enlistment. Following the exchange, Stewart was sent to the general rendezvous in Elmira, New York, to begin his military duties. Working in the ordnance section, Private Stewart performed in an acceptable fashion through early October.

His wanderlust was not quelled for long, however, and Private Stewart was tempted by an offer of promotion extended to him by Capt. David Jones, an officer in the 78th New York Volunteers. According to Stewart, Captain Jones offered him a position as his orderly sergeant. Apparently motivated by the promise of better pay and authority, in a rather brazen act Stewart, "deserted by donning the shoulder-straps, one day, and walking out past the guard, but was retaken on his way to Utica again."[3]

Capt. George L. Whiton of the 141st New York Volunteers, Private Stewart's commander, was neither amused nor impressed by this story. Desertion was an extremely serious offense that regrettably occurred too frequently. Any seasoned military leader could recount endless excuses proffered by captured deserters, and Private Stewart's version was no more credible than any other. As a consequence, Stewart found himself confined with four other prisoners in the guardhouse—barracks number three—to await a military tribunal that would decide his fate.

Private Stewart no doubt anxiously awaited his pending court-martial. Undoubtedly dominating his mind was his loss of freedom. He had never been confined before and the novel experience robbed him of his mobility. Always before, when threatened with discomfort, his fleet feet had brought him relief. Naturally, for Private Stewart, thoughts of escape took shape with every passing moment. What evolved was not a typical act born out of desperation but instead a well-calculated plot.

At the guardhouse an easy fraternity developed between the guards and the prisoners. Bound to each other day and night, the men's shared experience created common ground. Guards were not extensively trained in their duties and were often assigned guard duty from a roster of potential jobs. The line drawn between soldier–guard and soldier–prisoner was not defined by firm expectations, and the camaraderie combined with blurred boundaries occasionally produced disastrous outcomes. Good behavior earned rewards. Prisoners who complied with the simple guardhouse rules avoided rough treatment. One benefit that might accrue was a pass, which would break the tedium of seclusion for both the guard and the inmate.

Naturally, prisoners escorted into town were considered escape risks, and adequate precautions were taken to minimize the occurrence of escape. The ratio of guards to inmates favored security, and guards were cautioned to be on the alert for signs of intended escape.

With that focus, there was no suspicion raised when Private Stewart casually sauntered into two different drugstores and asked both druggists, "What are the effects of morphine?"[4] They each told him that vomiting and impaired sleep were the principle side effects and the drug was typically administered to relieve pain. Apparently satisfied with their response, Stewart purchased a small quantity of morphine.

The day following the trip to town heralded a fateful series of events.[5] Launching a well-calculated plot, Private Stewart proposed an evening of good whiskey drinking, and his fellow inmates gladly imbibed. Unbeknownst to the guards, who willingly participated in the alcohol social, Stewart had laced the whiskey with the previously acquired morphine. All drank freely, except Stewart, who carefully limited his consumption. This celebration was followed by a small epidemic of illness. Two people shook off the ill effects after copious vomiting, but, unfortunately, two others died—one only a few hours after drinking the morphine-whiskey concoction; the other, a day later.

An investigation was immediately launched following the deaths in barracks number three. Incriminating evidence, in the form of a bottle of liquor and two packages of a white substance, were recovered from Stewart's cell. The authorities were intent on proving Private Stewart's complicity. To that end, the stomach contents of one of the victims, along with the mysterious white powder seized from Private Stewart's cell, were forwarded to Professor Fowler of Geneva, New York, whose role was to analyze both and determine if there was a connection between the two.

The *Elmira Daily Gazette* reported the two deaths immediately. In complimentary tones that typified all future newspaper accounts, Private Stewart was described as "a young man of about twenty-two years of age, and has a mild, pleasant countenance . . . prepossessing and possessing more than ordinary talents. . . . He was about to have his trial by Court-martial, and undoubtedly sought to put a quietus on his guards, so that he could effect his escape, and by no means intended to administer a fatal dose."[6] The military took a more objective and determined approach, charging Pvt. Lorenzo Stewart with two counts of murder.

The *Elmira Daily Gazette* was either prescient or influential. Private Stewart's response to the criminal charges was to claim "nonintention to kill." His other line of defense was to claim insanity.

One of the more unusual aspects of this case was Private Stewart's access to legal assistance. His parents were described by the *Elmira Daily Gazette* as "very respectable people [who] reside in New York City." The newspaper reader was seemingly left to infer the high social standing Stewart's parents enjoyed.[7] It was, no doubt, Stewart's access to the wealth and influence of his parents that opened legal doors that remained closed to most military criminal defendants. A respected New York City law firm represented Private Stewart—his attorney was one F. B. Swift. Judge Advocate C. F. Young conducted the government prosecution. Private Stewart was charged with two major offenses: the double desertion and murder. The unusual nature of the crime and the caliber of Private Stewart's legal representation guaranteed a lengthy trial process. F. B. Swift, the consummate attorney, was thorough, thoughtful, and smart, which became immediately apparent as he began preparing his client's defense. Obtaining character witnesses was an early part of Swift's strategy. Before the trial began, he assembled witnesses from several cities around New York. As would any experienced attorney, Swift interviewed these potential witnesses and from their collective observations, he constructed a sympathetic portrait of his client.

Concede the obvious. Fortify the client's credibility. Build a story that both explains the misconduct and refutes the prosecution's version. These were the legal principles that guided Mr. Swift. To achieve those principles, he relied on exhaustive legal research, and his hard work was noticeable.

When the trial opened, Private Stewart immediately conceded his desertion from Rochester to become a substitute at Utica in early September 1863, but vigorously denied a prior enlistment and earlier desertion from the 14th Artillery at Ogdensburg, New York, in August. His abjuration was a challenge, and the military was forced to prove Stewart's complex travels, which ran from Rochester, to Ogdensburg, and ended in Utica; and involved two desertions, one from Rochester, which was admitted, and one from Ogdensburg, which was denied. The prosecution was not worried as they confidently countered Stewart's claims by presenting witnesses from the 14th Artillery. Unfortunately, soldiers from the 14th Artillery collectively equivocated and speculated that Stewart must have enlisted with the regiment in mid-August, thus undermining the prosecution's arguments. The testimony was timorous, unconvincing, and wholly disappointing. The officer who had enlisted Private Stewart cited poor memory; he could not recall the precise date that Stewart joined the regiment, again guessing sometime in August. The surgeon assigned the task of conducting Private Stewart's physical exam suffered a similar affliction. For Mr. Swift, the most satisfying revelation followed— Private Stewart's original enlistment papers had been lost. The prosecutor was humiliated, but despite these important tactical victories, Swift battled on. The defense called numerous witnesses, each one swearing that during the period of disputed enlistment Private Stewart had been an unencumbered civilian.

Disposing of the first accusation of desertion left yet another to refute, and the evidence indicting Private Stewart on this charge was stronger. Undermining the prosecution's evidence would not work as it had with the first charge; instead Private Stewart acknowledged that he freely left his unit. Stewart reminded the court of the "promised rewards for desertion thus held out to me by my superiors."[8] The implication was a subtle attack on the other regiment, an interesting ploy that shifted responsibility for misconduct away from Private Stewart, who could now claim status as a victim. Begging for mercy, Private Stewart appealed to each court member's sense of compassion. Succumbing to temptation was a human frailty. It represented weakness in response to seduction. A fair judgment would blame the deceiver and pity the deceived.

Private Stewart's legal defense of the two desertion charges was masterful. Murder was a different matter—this time, invoking a sympathetic response from the military court would be difficult, particularly since those who had died were soldiers. Swift probably concluded that the best approach was to admit the obvious. Deaths had occurred, and Private Stewart had been involved. Conceding the act of homicide allowed Swift to focus on Private Stewart's criminal intent. Throughout the trial, Private Stewart steadfastly claimed that the deaths had been accidental. His knowledge of medications was limited to that provided him by the druggists, and neither of them had mentioned that morphine was poisonous. Private Stewart admitted that he procured the morphine, but with the limited goal of inducing sleep to facilitate his escape. The story seemed plausible, and perhaps even Swift believed it. Whether Stewart's version was true or an elaborate falsehood, it nonetheless formed the core of his defense. Private Stewart deftly expressed this point with his impassioned closing plea to the court-martial members:

> The common law defines murder to be the willful taking of the life of another. The prosecution have failed to show any malice, any intent in regard to [the prison guards], or even a suspicion that I knew that morphine in any quantity would cause death, further than the question put to Dr. Tenny and his answer, which, to any but a person well acquainted with morphine, would leave the matter as vague as before. And I pray the Court to carefully examine into the probable motive for giving morphine to [the prison guards]; and if a doubt may arise in the mind of any member as to my guilt, for guilt can only arise from and be the effect of a wicked design—that I may receive the benefit of it and be judged in mercy accordingly. We are weak in our greatest strength. We are molded by circumstances, and the Court should carefully look to the incentives, the promised rewards for desertion thus held out to me by my superiors. . . . If the Court shall, on deliberating upon the Statements made by members of my own family, and upon the letters in evidence and Statements of letters I have been said to have written: and upon weighing them carefully, as taken in connection with my course in relation to which I am now being tried, If the Court shall determine that whether, owing to local permanent injury or to natural causes, there are periods when I am not responsible for my own acts, I pray the

Court to judge carefully and without prejudice in relation hereto, and herein also give me the benefit of any misgivings or doubts that may arise.[9]

On this note, the court-martial adjourned just before Christmas. The trial had consumed two weeks, an extraordinary length of time. After 240 pages of testimony had been recorded, the jury retired to deliberate. Private Stewart's eloquent closing plea distilled the essence of his defense: a lack of criminal intent to murder and frailty in submitting to proffered inducements to desert his regiment. Jury members probably misunderstood Stewart's comment alluding to "periods when I am not responsible for my own acts." Superficially, it seemed to be nothing more than a petition for mercy. In reality it was a craftily designed legal maneuver. Good attorneys like Swift imbedded different layers of arguments or legal exit strategies into their defense. If his client were denounced as guilty, these previously planted arguments would spring to life. This approach offered hope.

As Stewart awaited the verdict, the ever-faithful *Elmira Daily Gazette* swooned, "There will be considerable anxiety to learn his fate, and the public will wait impatiently until it is authoritatively announced."[10] As the newspaper regularly noted, Private Stewart had presented a credible defense. Numerous witnesses, including fellow soldiers, officers, and family members, all strode forth and supported his innocence. Swift provided expert legal assistance. Public opinion, at least as represented by the *Elmira Daily Gazette,* considered Private Stewart a victim of zealous military prosecution. Stewart was quietly confident, although his attorney was guarded.

A considerable period of time elapsed. Days turned into weeks, as the court-martial members reviewed the voluminous testimony. Some of Private Stewart's arguments seemed to make sense. He had challenged the claim regarding the desertion charges. Murder was more serious, but convincing testimony suggested that Private Stewart lacked criminal intent. Yes, Stewart had wished to escape by implementing his carefully devised plan. The deaths seemed to be the result of a terrible accident. Broken into pieces, Private Stewart's various misdeeds seemed to lose a malevolent cast. But when the military jury members reassembled his behavior, a different picture emerged and this picture was not flattering. Instead of an articulate, handsome victim, Private Stewart was seen as a conniving manipulator. These perceptions swirled around the accused, colliding with some basic facts. Two people were dead, two others had been made seriously ill. Private Stewart had joined an organization that rewarded submission—and punished opposition. Critical thinking was subordinated to blind compliance. The accused seemed too independent. The jury members might have studied Private Stewart's face closely. Doubt slowly eroded the mountain of defense-related testimony. Maybe Stewart was seen as too confident, even cavalier; he had shown no remorse or repentance. The jury had to weigh all these factors.

"All Hopes Gone," the *Elmira Daily Gazette* mournfully cried on April 21, 1864.[11] The commandant of the military post in Elmira delivered the sad, but now official word, to the breathless community. After thorough and thoughtful deliberation, the military jury had convicted Private Stewart, and their prescribed punishment was death. Military protocol required that all capital punishment be approved in Washington, D.C., and President Abraham Lincoln approved the sentence of death by hanging.[12] Following that early spring verdict, a guard of six men was posted outside barracks number three. Their mission was to ensure that neither escape nor suicide would thwart the will of military justice.

The bright spring days of April could do nothing to lighten Private Stewart's spirits; his mortal days on earth were limited. Stewart sat impassively with paper and pen in hand. His attorney, mindful of public opinion and the value of contrition, pushed for Stewart to pen a "confession."[13] From his barrack's cell, Private Stewart set about that gloomy task, perhaps thinking a public "confession" might yet reverse his fate.

In a firm hand, full of resolution, Private Stewart scribed a lengthy note. His declaration of guilt began on a pious note. Stewart praised his parents, who had prepared him for "life beyond the grave where all who are received by our Savior can live forever." The adulation continued, as Stewart described a heavenly childhood devoid of conflict and full of promise. In Private Stewart's public admission, a dark shadow was cast on his life when he left home to join the military. This dichotomy between good home life and bad military life was expressed in Private Stewart's characteristic eloquence. "From that time down to the present I have been tossed about upon the sea of life like a man upon a ship in the midst of the Atlantic."

Private Stewart's "confession" offered his public audience more information. Readers learned that his decision to enlist had been an economic one. In the months preceding his enlistment, Stewart had been trying his hand at entrepreneurship, but visions of a fast fortune faded as Stewart started selling magazine subscriptions "in our larger Cities." Buyers were scarce, and debts started piling up. According to Stewart, his landlady lost patience and demanded overdue rent payments; however, he didn't mention that she made any legal threats against him. It was no doubt humiliating for Stewart to plead poverty, but circumstances forced him to. The military offered the promise of a steady, albeit meager, paycheck. Although Stewart must have recognized his primary motivation to enter military service was financial, he nonetheless publicly proclaimed, "I resolved to enter the service of my Country and prove myself one of many who really are activated by motives of patriotism alone."

From this point forward, Stewart's confession contained few revelations. Stewart wrote that within a day or two of enlisting, he received a compelling offer from Capt. David Jones, 78th New York Volunteers. "Come be my orderly Sergeant," Captain Jones had purportedly intoned; however, the officer had been unable to effect Stewart's transfer. At his trial, Private Stewart insisted that when he deserted he had obtained permission to leave camp.

Private Stewart completed the handwritten confession, and it was conveyed to the local newspaper and promptly printed. The editorial accompaniment was predictable. The *Elmira Daily Gazette* was unshrinking in solicitude, "Notwithstanding the enormity of his crime, he has the sympathy of the community, and in requesting the prayers of all Christians for his soul's welfare, exhibits a contrition of spirit, which he has manifested for the last few days of his confinement."[14]

Private Stewart surely monitored his press coverage. Following the editorial comments accompanying his confession, Stewart felt compelled to respond. Writing to the editor of the *Elmira Daily Gazette*, Private Stewart took exception to a description rendering him as "being indifferent." "I am represented as appearing to be 'indifferent to the fate that awaits me.' I am sorry if anything I have said or done since my sentence has produced such an impression."[15]

Private Stewart likely retained a flicker of hope that was nurtured by the sympathetic public reaction. The reporters of the *Elmira Daily Gazette* never expressed any doubt. If cynicism had ever crept into the public psyche, twisted by a suspicion that their sentiments had been manipulated by a clever legal defense strategy, Private Stewart would have suffered a loss of support, but, apparently, that never occurred. Emboldened by the compassionate community response, Stewart's next step was easy. Even the post commandant may have encouraged his next letter—a direct appeal for clemency to President Abraham Lincoln.

The letter President Lincoln examined was well crafted. Stewart confidently quoted a cast of character references. The post commandant (as were other officers) was "well aware that I am not guilty of deliberate murder and wishes me to be dealt with justly. . . . All I ask is a thorough investigation of the case and if any sensible and unprejudiced man can find me guilty from the testimony then I deserve death."[16]

Lincoln, the wise attorney and embattled president, was probably uneasy about the potential insanity issue. There had been no shortage of testimony or competent legal representation at Stewart's trial, but scattered throughout the transcripts were bothersome indications of "periods when I [Stewart] am not responsible for my own acts." Nowhere in the transcripts did expert medical testimony touch on this nettlesome issue. The President chose a cautious stance. To execute a man who might lack the sensibilities to understand punishment ran counter to civilized mores. Only one reasonable option existed. President Lincoln stayed the execution and ordered a medical inquiry into Private Stewart's mental state.

It seemed like a storybook drama. One day before the planned hanging, Private Stewart received his precious reprieve.[17] President Lincoln had communicated his request to Assistant Adjutant General E. D. Townsend. The President's desire was quickly converted to an official order.

Maj. Gen. John A. Dix, Commanding the Department of the East, and Col. Seth Eastman at Elmira were the recipients of Townsend's action. Fortunately, the directive was transmitted by telegraph. On April 21, Stewart's execution was suspended. The *Elmira Daily Gazette* breathed a sigh of relief. "The sympathies of all have been interested in his behalf, which when the news of the suspension of his sentence was received, manifested itself by expressions of joy which could not be misunderstood other than friendly."[18]

Stewart must have been ecstatic. The stay of execution vindicated, at least temporarily, the juggernaut of inequity that threatened his death. The pause allowed both attorney and client to recover from their harrowing experience. During this brief interlude, Private Stewart's attorney carefully studied President Lincoln's order. It was clear that the next step required a physician's evaluation of the defendant. The medical inquiry was conducted through the formality of a special commission.[19] In this case, the commission consisted of one member, Dr. John P. Gray, a respected physician at the Utica Insane Asylum. Close, frequent exposure to individuals suffering from various degrees of debilitating mental disorders made Dr. Gray an excellent choice for evaluating Private Stewart.

Dr. Gray's medical inquiry bore much procedural similarity to a court-martial. That procedural authority was tied in with the special commission status granted the investigation. As a consequence, the medical inquiry was essentially an adversarial process. Both the prosecutor and the defense counsel subjected any evidence developed by Dr. Gray to scrutiny. Both sides, together with Dr. Gray, would take testimony from witnesses, and all witness statements were captured in a verbatim written record.

Private Stewart was almost certainly apprehensive; his best hope sprang from the possibility that family members, fellow soldiers, and the medical examination would confirm he was unsound of mind. The prosecution, however, might successfully counter his claim of insanity, in which case, Private Stewart's reprieve would be short-lived. Reinstatement of the death penalty would be the price for failure.

Dr. Gray wasted no time in assembling the inquiry. The witnesses were made immediately available, and the stage was set to gather evidence toward the end of April 1864. Dr. Gray began the process by conducting a personal examination of Stewart on April 29 and 30.[20]

Private Stewart's "revelations" to Dr. Gray consisted almost entirely of an opus of innocence. Repeatedly, Stewart stressed his complete lack of malevolent intent. The failed transfer to Captain Jones's regiment was a bitter pill to swallow, Private Stewart explained, and his arrest was humiliating. Anger consumed his mind, breeding thoughts of escape.

Dr. Gray took careful notes, as he skillfully directed the interview. It was important to hear the accused soldier account for the deaths. Private Stewart explained, "I went, with my guard, into Mr. Mead's drug store in Elmira to buy some segars [sic] on an order from some of the prisoners who could not get into town."[21] This innocent expedition had planted the seed for an innovative escape, and Private Stewart had wasted no time harvesting his bounty.

Private Stewart reported that he had casually entered the drugstore and gazed about, observing several people, among them Dr. Tenny. The real aim of his interest, though, had been a small bottle labeled "morphia." Private Stewart telegraphed his familiarity with the drug's characteristics by declaring to Dr. Gray, "I was at once struck with an idea and without loss of a moment I began its execution."

Private Stewart said he had quizzed Mr. Mead and Dr. Tenny about the effects of an overdose of morphia, and neither of them had hesitated in answering. Both agreed that vomiting and disturbed sleep were the chief effects of an overdose. Private Stewart quietly purchased an ounce of the soporific and admitted he was astonished at the ease with which he was able to do it. No one had even questioned the purchase of morphia by a jailed soldier![22]

Private Stewart reported that he had breathed a quiet sigh of relief when he left the drugstore. His escorts returned him to the barracks and since, "whiskey was always for sale at the barracks . . . I purchased a pint . . . ,"[23] which he promptly but discreetly mixed with the morphia.

But, Private Stewart admitted, he had made a mistake. Part of his devious plot was observed by a fellow prisoner who watched Stewart hide the bottle of whiskey. Stewart could only guess that the bystander had drawn the conclusion that he had hidden the whiskey to avoid having to share it, which violated customs of behavior among inmates. Apparently thirst, desire, and injustice were stimuli too great for the other inmate to resist, and when Private Stewart left the area, his fellow inmate had stolen the whiskey. Unfortunately, he had not seen Private Stewart lace the whiskey with the morphia, and he drank freely, completely oblivious to the danger.

Private Stewart reported that he had been alarmed when he later sought to retrieve his poisoned whiskey and discovered it missing. A desperate search discovered the sodden culprit. There was still some whiskey left. Relieved, Private Stewart reclaimed his treasure. "I put the bottle in my pocket and when at work offered the drink to the guards."[24]

Amazingly, none of the four guards were rendered unconscious. A couple vomited and all told Stewart the whiskey tasted bitter. Disappointed, Stewart grudgingly returned to the guardhouse.

His disappointment was replaced by fear later that night. One of the guards died, along with the unwitting prisoner who had stolen the whiskey. Word of Private Stewart's complicity spread like wildfire though the barracks. Anger followed quickly on its heels, and a lynching party was proposed. Were it not for the intervention of the night officer of the guard, Private Stewart's story would surely have ended more abruptly.

Dr. Gray probably impressed all members of the medical inquiry. He was no doubt serious in purpose and organized in approach, and a certain quiet confidence accompanied his style, which must have been comforting to witnesses, as he interviewed them. Private Stewart's mother was particularly hesitant. She appeared to be nervous, no doubt intimidated by the process, but the physician soothed her anxiety.

Private Stewart's mother had a powerful voice. Her former uncertainty at testifying dissipated rapidly. Clearly, her son's life was at stake. Through the gentle structure framed by Private Stewart's attorney, her story unfolded.[25]

Leroy, as Private Stewart's mother had christened him, had been an unusual child. Perhaps, his affliction resulted from a childhood head injury, or maybe, his mother wondered aloud, the sunstroke he had suffered as a teenager was the culprit. "He has been subject to these singular attacks . . . I was fearful he would not be able to do any business."

Taking the cue, Dr. Gray probed for further details of the attacks, and Private Stewart's mother eagerly described one of many she had witnessed. "When he was about seven years old he came in and sat down at the dinner table. . . . He looked at the plate for a moment and then got up and went from the table. His father asked him to come back . . . and he made no answer. He then went out of the room . . . and finally we found him in the sitting room fast asleep under the table cover." Alarmed by this midday fit of sleepiness, Private Stewart's father attempted to rouse his son. When that failed, he carried the sleepy child to his bed, where he slept until the next day. When he did arise he was confused and physically weak. Stewart's parents were confused but felt helpless to intervene.

These strength-sapping fits painted only part of the picture. Private Stewart was a moody person. As his mother frequently observed, "He would appear melancholy and walk the floor with his hands in his pockets. Very frequently when he would be in that way and would not get violent he would lay down and go to sleep." Again a lengthy period of somnolence was followed by confusion on awakening.

Over time, additional evidence of mental instability emerged. His mother described Private Stewart's blithe outlook on personal belongings. "He was always giving away all his own things. He never placed any value on money or clothes." A bit more ominous was his tendency to pilfer items. Private Stewart's mother quickly modified her description of the behavior. There seemed to be no conceivable reason why certain items were stolen. On one occasion, Private Stewart took a currycomb from a local store. His parents were baffled—they didn't own a horse. Many such items mysteriously appeared. Although suspicious, Stewart's parents were inclined to accept his habitual response. "He would insist that he didn't know anything . . . just such things were happening all his life."

Private Stewart's adolescence ushered in a new phase. Itchy feet took over, and, for weeks on end, he would disappear from home. Returning home from one such excursion in 1861, Private Stewart surprised his family with a plan to get married. Private Stewart's mother reacted with some ambivalence. She reported thinking that perhaps marriage would have a settling influence on Leroy. But, driven by unease, Stewart's mother felt compelled to caution "his wife before she married him, and told her everything in reference to his peculiarities and that he was not a fit subject to be married." Despite this warning, love prevailed, and Stewart married on September 5, 1861.

The honeymoon would be three or four weeks, Private Stewart had proudly declared. The newlyweds left midweek for their special time together, but to the surprise of everyone, they returned home in a few days. Neither of them answered the questions asked by perplexed family members. After being at home for two weeks, Stewart left them all for "business in Toledo." Private Stewart's mother dramatically concluded her testimony at this point.

The patriarch of the family was the next person summoned by Dr. Gray.[26] Private Stewart's father extended the history signifying a pattern of mental instability. "He was silly. He didn't care who was present and what he said."

Private Stewart had a temper, too. Gray developed this line of investigation, directing a question to Stewart's father: "You say he threatened to shoot you on one occasion." Stewart's father bristled.

Apparently those were painful memories that had been long since buried.

Stewart's father did confirm one peculiar habit: Leroy frequently pilfered items from local merchants. The shop owners grew familiar with Stewart's routine and accommodated it by making an informal arrangement between them and Stewart's parents. When Stewart took items from the shops, the shop owners prepared a bill, and Private Stewart's family regularly received and promptly paid these bills.

Private Stewart was a wonderful storyteller, and generally he used this talent to serve some attempt at deception. Not all shop owners were willing to overlook Stewart's bad behavior. Those who took offense at his casual approach to their property were subjected to Stewart's classic deceit. "Sometimes he said another boy took them and he didn't, and sometimes he wanted it for this purpose and sometimes for that purpose." Private Stewart's father admitted there were countless similar examples.

Private Stewart's sister had listened while her parents described Leroy. Now it was her turn. She was able to confirm many of the observations provided by her parents. She described one incident in particular that seemed to capture her brother's bizarre behavior:

On one of his extended excursions, Stewart had written a passionate letter to his sister.[27] According to the letter, the boarding house where he was staying had burned down, and all of his worldly possessions had been destroyed. Private Stewart's sister testified, "He wrote me that he was entirely destitute, and I supposed that he was." The concern motivated by Stewart's letter impelled her to assemble a package of necessities and mail it to him.

Eventually Stewart's sister learned the real story. Perhaps a lifelong distrust of her brother had bred skepticism. "We found out subsequently that the fire had never occurred, and that he had not lost an article." When Private Stewart returned home, he stepped into a briar patch. Prickly family members demanded an explanation. No doubt frustrated, but surely not surprised, Stewart's family listened incredulously. "He denied having written the account of the fire." To compound the mystery, Private Stewart denied ever receiving his sister's care package.

Stewart's attorney, family, and Dr. Gray's pointed questions illustrated an unbalanced mind. Their collective renderings portrayed a person ridden by impulsive acts, bouts of pervasive melancholy, "fits," excessive somnolence, confusion, a careless concern about theft, aimless wanderings, and thoughtless mendacity. Left unchallenged, this testimony was no doubt persuasive.

The government prosecutor naturally cross-examined each of Private Stewart's witnesses. After the defense exhausted their witness list, Dr. Gray heard testimony from the prosecution. The prosecutor was determined to prove that Private Stewart was sane.

Campbell Young was a familiar face to Private Stewart.[28] He had been the successful prosecutor from the court-martial, and now, he was a witness at the medical inquiry. "Have you seen the prisoner since the trial?" queried Capt. C. C. Barton, the current judge advocate. "Yes," Young replied, "It was perhaps within five or six days or a week after the sentence was read to him. . . . He expressed regrets at having to suffer a violent death for a crime which he did not think he had been guilty of." The intent of this testimony was to cast doubt. If Private Stewart was mentally ill, there had been no hint of instability as he faced the stress of his conviction. Quite the contrary—Campbell Young described Stewart as firmly in control of his emotions.

A minister, Isaac Clark, testified for the prosecution.[29] This was a shrewd maneuver. During his long confinement, Private Stewart often sought spiritual comfort. It never occurred to him that his words would be used to indict him. The minister had probably encouraged a frank, uncensored exchange. Neither Dr. Gray nor the defense counsel apparently raised a legal objection to this breach of confidence. That permitted Clark the unrestricted opportunity to discuss intimate revelations. Clark acknowledged a total of three visits to console Private Stewart. The preacher's testimony benefited from a double credibility boost, the integrity expected from a man of the cloth and the truthfulness of the confessor. The judge advocate asked a simple question. "Did you observe anything in his manner different from what you would observe in any person under similar circumstances?" Isaac Clark's response was simple and direct, "No, Sir."

Stewart's attorney tried to undermine the minister's testimony. The principle strategy employed was to criticize, indirectly, the amount of time the pair shared together. "What was the length of your third interview?" Swift demanded. "Not more than fifteen minutes because it was just before his dinner hour," the minister responded.

Whatever points the attorneys scored were imperceptible. Throughout the proceedings, Dr. Gray remained impassive. After all witnesses were heard, the inquiry was finished on May 7, 1864. Private Stewart, his attorney, and Stewart's family awaited the results of the medical inquiry.

A veritable mountain of information awaited Dr. Gray's analysis. His final medical opinion incorporated the court-martial evidence, testimony from the medical inquiry, and the direct examination of Stewart. Six days after completing the medical inquiry into Private Stewart's sanity, Dr. Gray submitted his report to President Lincoln.

President Lincoln carefully reviewed the medical report from his Special Commissioner, Dr. Gray. Dr. Gray's intelligence, thoroughness, and wisdom were amply represented in the report, which summarized important events in Private Stewart's life and touched on the head injury Stewart suffered at the age of five and the sunstroke when he was a teenager. Dr. Gray conjectured that as a consequence of these injuries a constellation of symptoms resulted. Mental delirium was the central symptom, around which rotated headaches, drowsiness, and frequent nosebleeds.[30]

Dr. Gray had studied several letters authored by Private Stewart as part of his evaluation and became convinced that an examination of Stewart's uncensored written thoughts might reveal his inner feelings, from which two trends emerged. Clearly, Private Stewart was a dreamer. His letters outlined fantastic, improbable get-rich ideas, some of which were on the verge of being irrational. A different trend was apparent when Stewart authored patently false statements. Some were apparently designed to elicit sympathy; others intended for selfish gain. The puzzle for Dr. Gray was determining whether Private Stewart was insane or simply a fraud who manipulated people for his own needs. Judging by the quality of his letters, there was little doubt that Private Stewart was intelligent. He was bright, well schooled, and an avid reader.

Dr. Gray felt it necessary to address Private Stewart's proclivity toward violence. Evidence had surfaced during the medical inquiry suggesting tendencies in that direction. In spite of the fact that testimony from Stewart's father indicated Stewart had a history of acting out, Dr. Gray said he could not reach a firm conclusion. The best he could offer, based on the limited evidence, was a suspicion that Private Stewart might become violent with sufficient provocation. Part of Gray's concern might have been based on Stewart's seeming disdain for authority. Private Stewart had often vented his displeasure with (corrupt) military leaders. "Hundreds of officers were put in commission through influence at court, wealth or personal influence deciding appointments that should have been made solely on the basis of merit."[31]

In his report, Dr. Gray gave great weight to the observations of Stewart's physician, Dr. Woodward. As a professional colleague, his insights were particularly valuable concerning the presence of a mental delirium, and establishing that diagnosis was critical to a determination of insanity. Dr. Woodward had treated Private Stewart during one of his most severe fits of delirium. "This young man's nervous system was highly susceptible to impressions. . . . The delirium was ephemeral, not peculiar, in character, and subsided rapidly and entirely. The phenomena had not the exaggeration, force, intensity, and delusional character and persistency of a maniacal paroxysm. He had no recollection of occurrences during this period, which is common in delirium."

The report submitted to President Lincoln was a model of evenhandedness. Facts were presented in such a manner that any reader could objectively judge the case. Rhetorical arguments, either supporting or disproving insanity, were provided. A useful report nonetheless had to answer the ultimate question: Was Private Stewart insane? Dr. Gray finally concluded that the numerous examples of wrongdoing attributed to Private Stewart did not "upon a close scrutiny of each and all of them, exhibit a sufficient want of reasonable motive, nor a sufficient absence of the power of self-control, to indicate the presence of insanity."

Dr. Gray reached his final opinion after considering three medical disorders often associated with insanity. Those three were delirium, mania, and delusions. Each was discussed in turn. Using each diagnosis as a template, Dr. Gray compared Private Stewart's history. With each comparison, symptoms were lacking. As a result, Dr. Gray rejected Private Stewart's contention that he had suffered a lifelong mental illness.

The medical report focused next on the murders attributed to Private Stewart. Dr. Gray reflected on the poisoning, and, striking a balanced note, conceded that both sane and insane behaviors were present. Perhaps a brief episode of insanity intruded on Stewart's mind and caused his misbehavior. A thoughtful medical-legal opinion demanded a careful review of Private Stewart's mental state before, during, and after the crime. Dr. Gray's examination of witnesses was designed in part to tease out that chronology. In a similar fashion, his interview of Private Stewart sought to identify any trace of a mental disorder, past or present. This methodical approach left no doubt in Dr. Gray's mind concerning Private Stewart's sanity.

Dr. Gray bolstered his determination of sanity through oblique references to Stewart's malingering. "He appreciated readily my questions, and answered without reserve, except when an answer would criminate himself, or tend to degrade his character." According to Gray, Stewart demonstrated selective memory deficits when he uniformly forgot potentially embarrassing information. As the pattern grew more obvious, Dr. Gray's skepticism deepened. "Such want of consciousness of wrong acts, whether criminal or mischievous, is not consistent with this clear knowledge and remembrance of wrong acts," reported Dr. Gray. Only the rational mind could consistently identify risk in certain responses and adapt accordingly.

Both family and defense counsel had sought to convince Dr. Gray that Private Stewart was impulsive and irrational. The argument ultimately failed because the doctor was impressed by the self-control Stewart possessed in so many different settings.

Private Stewart benefited from an almost unprecedented review. His court-martial was fully litigated. Numerous witnesses testified for both sides. Following the conviction, Stewart had rallied public interest sufficiently to have the President of the United States intervene. By his order, a respected physician conducted a medical inquiry. To Private Stewart's chagrin, Dr. Gray resolved that he was entirely sane.

Dr. Gray considered Stewart eccentric. The diagnosis of eccentricity spanned the gap between insanity and normality. The term was a popular one advanced by the emerging discipline of phrenology which claimed an impressive crowd of professional adherents. German physician Franz Joseph Gall developed the theory and medical research on the subject was regularly reported in a popular journal of phrenology. Phrenology proposed that a structural-functional model for the human brain existed. According to the theory, thirty-seven distinct areas in the brain controlled behavior. Some were considered well matched to human emotions like hope or destructiveness. These thirty-seven areas of the brain corresponded with similar regions on a person's skull. Detailed maps were developed that guided the diagnostician across the bumps and valleys of the subject's head, and careful analysis of the bumps and valleys unlocked the person's character. Phrenologists contended that the various bumps on a person's skull collectively predicted human behavior. They would carefully inspect a person's skull and diagnose mental aberrations. Eccentricity was diagnosed when a specific pattern of skull protuberances was identified. Phrenologists equated eccentricity with excessive individuality, high intelligence, and emotional indifference.[32]

A different concept of eccentricity focused on the weak judgment, vacillating emotions, and whimsical lifestyle experienced by the sufferer. "A very curious form of impaired mind is now and then met with in individuals, who, without any particular want of principle, and often without any assignable motive, are disposed to exaggerate every-thing . . . which interferes with the truth of what they narrate; a dispo-sition to indulge the imagination, combined with an indifference to fact and reality. . . ," authoritatively intoned a medical description appended by Dr. Gray to his medical report. President Lincoln accepted Dr. Gray's conclusion. Many months would pass before Pri-vate Stewart learned the outcome.

The case of *United States v. Lorenzo Stewart* is like a time capsule. Opening the capsule many years later reveals a rare piece of Ameri-can Civil War history. Inside is a fully litigated court-martial docu-menting an insanity defense. Military jurisprudence was an essential, often neglected part of the Civil War saga. The military law set impor-tant boundaries, and transgressors were judged and punished accord-ingly. Specific legal procedures ensured, at least in principle, a fair trial. Military law recognized humanitarian considerations, and one of these was mental illness. When the war began, mental illness was a crude, distant consideration. The massive mobilization undertaken to wage war forced an intense reexamination of human behavior. This was driven by the need to recruit, retain, and control the influx of men. As the war dragged on, the emotional toll attracted the attention of some military leaders and physicians. A new spectrum of non-battle-related conditions, such as a pathologic homesickness, emerged, and they affected alarming numbers of soldiers. To accom-modate these emotional casualties of war, special facilities were erected.

Private Stewart undertook a relatively rare legal defense—insanity—to escape punishment. Other misbehaving soldiers, more seriously afflicted with mental symptoms, were acquitted by reason of insanity and were involuntarily committed to mental institutions for treatment. F. B. Swift, the attorney representing Private Stewart, must have considered other outcomes. His client, for example, faced either execution or a lengthy prison term if convicted. An effective defense required legal research. Swift reviewed military law, the appellate process, actual courts-martial cases, and the military prison system. Private Stewart's story was complicated by medical testimony, which required Swift to become familiar with a wide array of emotional disorders. To educate himself, Swift probably developed an extensive collection of papers. His filing system would have needed only three labels: madness, malingering, and malfeasance.

CHAPTER TWO

MILITARY MALFEASANCE

P vt. Lorenzo Stewart held membership in a select group. Courts-martial for serious felonies were rare. Whether the victim was military or civilian, the military reserved the option to prosecute serious acts of malfeasance. *Military malfeasance* is a broad term encompassing the typical felonies like murder, theft, and rape, along with crimes unique to the military, such as desertion, disobeying orders, and mutiny. Prosecuting their own served notice on other troops while reassuring civilians that military personnel were accountable and controllable. Given the gravity of Private Stewart's murder trial, his attorney would have prepared by studying actual military capital cases. The attorney must understand what crimes, and most importantly what aggravating features, contribute to a death penalty. Was accidentally killing a military guard sufficient? Did desertion, coupled with an escape plan, justify execution? Was the military dominated by the philosophy, "Pardon one offense, and you encourage the commission of many"?[1]

According to official records, approximately forty-five executions were performed each year from the time the Civil War began. The types of offenses receiving the ultimate punishment were fairly limited.

The vast majority of known death penalty verdicts followed standard courts-martial procedures. This afforded the accused at least some safeguards, such as an established, albeit weak, appeal process.

Two official executions resulted from drumhead courts-martial, which are courts-martial that try offenses on the battlefield, sacrificing a full legal due process for expedience. The goal was rapid disposition of criminal charges. The accusers no doubt believed the evidence justified this approach. The victims in both cases were soldiers apprehended and accused of desertion. Unfortunately, justice was the ultimate casualty of this approach. Unofficial drumhead proceedings were recorded in diaries and letters, suggesting the practice was slightly more common than officially recognized. Clearly as military justice evolved, the balance between fairness, expediency, and deterrence demanded that individual legal rights be afforded greater protection. Unfortunately, before the balance was reset, an untold number of soldiers suffered the ultimate penalty.[2]

Charles Humphreys was a chaplain assigned to the 2nd Massachusetts Cavalry, who served two masters: his military commanders and God.[3] On a day-to-day basis, a chaplain was a comforting presence. For the most part it was a predictable life. A chaplain generally accompanied the regiment into battle, armed only with his religious beliefs, and the soldiers invited his informal counsel. Some chaplains supplemented the Sabbath service with Bible study or prayer meetings.

Chaplain Humphreys was no firebrand. Through a quiet display of his faith, he earned the respect of both officers and troops. He accurately calculated that fiery sermonizing would paradoxically extinguish the faith he sought to kindle. On Sunday, he would preach from any makeshift pulpit.

In general, chaplains were a versatile lot, and whenever comfort and commiseration was needed, a chaplain ministered. Common services might include a prayer before battle, succor to a wounded soldier, or relief from the torment of homesickness. The advice chaplains routinely offered did not extend to legal matters, unless plaintively requested by a condemned soldier.

Chaplain Humphreys recalled, "The hardest duty that ever fell to my lot as chaplain was to prepare a deserter to die."[4] Compounding the discomfort was Humphreys' familiarity with the soldier.

The drumhead court-martial was convened shortly after the Massachusetts soldier was arrested. His apprehension followed a skirmish with a band of Southern guerrillas. The soldier had enlisted in the Union Army but cast aside his allegiance, to join the enemy. Desertion was bad enough but taking up arms against the Union was fatal. The captured turncoat asked Chaplain Humphreys to represent him at the drumhead court-martial, and Humphreys agreed. Opposing Humphreys was a skilled prosecutor; Lewis Dabney was the judge advocate, a position earned by his prosecutorial skill. Dabney's compelling rhetoric, combined with the facts of the case, sealed the soldier's fate. Humphreys interjected two mitigating factors: the soldier's youth and his seducement by a southern woman. The predetermined pronouncement of guilt was formalized by the field trial, and the soldier was sentenced to death. No mercy would intervene between verdict and punishment.

"The poor victim chose to lean on my arm as he walked to execution behind his own coffin borne by his old messmates, while the band marched beside playing a funeral dirge. And he leaned still more closely on my faith."[5]

Chaplain Humphreys escorted the condemned soldier to his place of execution. Just before his eyes were bound with a handkerchief, the soldier pleaded with his fellow soldiers. "Comrades! I want to acknowledge that I am guilty and that my punishment is just . . . take warning from my example, and whatever comes do not desert the old flag for which I am proud to die."[6]

Humphreys shook hands with the soldier, offering a final earthly tribute. With unbelievable composure, the soldier sat on his coffin and loudly proclaimed, "I am ready." The six-man firing squad responded obligingly and dispatched the soldier to the hereafter.

A properly constituted court-martial was governed by stricter rules. Imposition of the death penalty required concurrence from two-thirds of the courts-martial members. Two crimes led the list of those officially recorded as being punished by execution: desertion and murder.

The official list of U.S. soldiers executed between 1861 and 1866 records the names of 267 men. There were no officers on the list; the vast majority of those executed had never advanced beyond the rank of private. Two first sergeants jointly shared the "honor" of holding the highest rank among those executed. Fifty-two soldiers executed were former members of the U.S. Colored Troops, New York troops accounted for thirty-five, Connecticut twenty-four, and Pennsylvania twenty-three. More than half of those executed suffered that fate after deserting, while another quarter were convicted of murder. Less than 10 percent were executed for rape or mutiny, and a surprisingly small group was convicted of stealing or espionage.[7]

Among the U.S. Colored Troops twenty-seven were convicted of murder, fourteen of mutiny, and ten for rape. Only one was executed for desertion. Two-thirds of New York troops who suffered the death penalty were convicted of desertion, and five were convicted of murder. All but two Connecticut troops were executed for desertion. That same pattern was duplicated with Pennsylvania soldiers: Eighteen deserted and five were convicted as murderers.[8]

The Articles of War had many references to unauthorized absences. Article 22 directed that "No noncommissioned officer or soldier shall enlist himself in any other regiment, troop, or company, without a regular discharge . . . on the penalty of being a deserter, and suffer accordingly."[9]

Article 20 set forth the penalty for desertion: "All officers and soldiers who have received pay, or have been duly enlisted in the service of the United States and shall be convicted of having deserted the same, shall suffer death, or such other punishment as, by sentence of a court-martial, shall be inflicted."[10]

Initially, Article 20 allowed some discretion in determining the punishment for desertion; however, an act of Congress removed all ambiguity in 1861. Henceforth, any conviction for desertion during a time of war demanded, without discretion, the imposition of the death penalty. The only other military crime afforded this dubious distinction was forcing a safeguard, which was a directed order to protect an enemy. Forcing a safeguard violated this military order that was issued to the protected party.

Court-martial practice permitted the jury members two choices for a condemned soldier: hanging or a firing squad. Clearly the firing squad was preferred—two-thirds chose that option. The sentence was generally orchestrated to leave a searing impression on the spectators. An entire division might be assembled to watch an execution. Troops were arranged in a large rectangle with one end left open. A double column of soldiers created a corridor, through which the prisoner and his procession marched. The provost marshal led the spectacle, followed by a band, an armed guard, the coffin, prisoner, chaplain, and another armed guard. Bringing up the rear were twelve men who would deliver the final punishment. To ensure success, an additional reserve of six men was prepared to carry out the execution, if for any reason the designated group failed. This "death march" was designed to both humiliate the prisoner and chill the observers.[11] The extent to which the latter succeeded was debatable.

"I have just this moment arrived from witnessing the execution of a soldier of the 5th Maine regiment for desertion," Daniel M. Holt, a surgeon, wrote to his wife. The surgeon described to his wife the criminal's last moments. "The prisoner seated upon his coffin, while different bands composing the division strike up a dirge as he slowly moves along, until at length arriving at the fatal spot, the vehicle stops, he is helped to dismount—the coffin is taken out and placed upon the ground while he sits upon it listening to the reading of the findings of the court and death warrant; a prayer by the Chaplain, binding the eyes and upon a signal given, eight bullets pierce the heart and the spirit goes to meet its God." According to the surgeon's letter, the drama left an indelible impression on him. He indicated that he fervently hoped he would never witness another execution and that such a disgrace would never dishonor his own family.[12]

Pvt. John D. Billings, a member of the 10th Battery, Massachusetts Light Artillery, witnessed several executions.[13] The hideous affairs led this onlooker to a different conclusion. "I do not believe that the shooting of a deserter had any great deterring influence on the rank and file; for the opportunities to get away safely were most abundant." This was a setback for a military prevention strategy that miscalculated the impact of an execution on battle-hardened troops.

The twelve soldiers detached to form the firing unit faced the accused as he sat on his coffin. Eleven of the twelve weapons were loaded with real ammunition, and one held a blank cartridge. In this way, none of the members of the firing squad could be sure that his was the fatal bullet. The rifle squad was ordered to take careful aim and fire. Each spectator filed past the corpse, perhaps offering a final silent tribute, an experience that no doubt was observed with mixed emotions.

Most executions were carried out flawlessly and the drama unfolded as expected, which probably left most observers satisfied that justice had been fairly dispensed. The prisoner paid the ultimate penalty—quickly and with limited suffering. Bungled executions affected witnesses in a different way, diverting their attention from justice being served to the prisoner's anguish. The original purpose for the punishment was lost in the prisoner's death struggle. In a twist of fate, the perpetrator became the victim.

The memory of injustice was occasionally recorded in the diaries of witnesses. In one example, John M. Hawkes, a surgeon, reported in 1864 that: "Sgt. Walker Co. A, 3rd S. C. Inf. [Union, colored] was shot by sentence of court martial at 10:00 A.M. . . . 5 balls entered the body, one the head. Two vollies were fired 12 paces off. At first the culprit staggered back one pace & fell. I examined his wounds briefly and retired and the other volley was fired as he lay on the ground."[14]

Mass executions were just as unpleasant. The spectacle of several men facing death together epitomized military efficiency and minimized disruptions to camp life. Organizing the troops for multiple executions, though, was a challenge. The risk of blunders increased with the complicated choreography.

A group of five deserters from the 1st Connecticut Heavy Artillery faced their fate together near Laurel Hill, Virginia, on December 21,

1864. A sixty-man firing unit divided into five equal sections was organized. The field was jam-packed with prisoners, executioners, and
witnesses. At the appointed time, the prisoners were separated, and
each rifle squad aimed down its narrow zone. A centrally placed officer barked his command: "Fire!" Amazingly, after the deafening
retort, not one person was felled. The prisoners were stunned.
Alarmed, but prepared, the large reserve unit moved forward and
fired, immediately killing three prisoners, but only wounding the
other two. The provost marshal was unwavering. While others were
no doubt sickened by the affair, he removed his revolver and shot the
struggling survivors. One determined soul still resisted, and the resolute provost moved up and put a bullet through the brain of the last
survivor.[15]

The military desperately sought a means to control the flight of
deserters. Once again, the military struggled to strike a balance
between preserving the fighting force and maintaining legal protection for an accused soldier. This was a delicate exercise, which, if
crudely conducted, would erode public support for the military. Many
years would pass before one glaring omission was corrected—the
absence of a military appointed defense counsel. For the most part
soldiers were left to defend themselves—an unequal battle, pitting an
accused enlisted soldier against a prosecuting officer.

Pvt. William I. Lynch, Company B, 63rd New York Volunteers,
was unquestionably a bold rogue. Private Lynch was a talented escape
artist who flirted with death. His tendency to roam surfaced early in
the war, to the consternation of his military unit. Disgruntled members of his company were the first to track him down, and when they
did, he was promptly arrested. His unauthorized sojourn resulted in
his confinement at the Albany Barracks, from which Lynch was to
escape at least three times. The regiment Lynch was assigned to was
eventually deployed, and their prisoner would not accompany them.
Private Lynch was transferred to David's Island, New York, in the
summer of 1862, and he escaped from there as well.[16]

This time, several months passed before Private Lynch was apprehended in September 1862. His capture was worth a five-dollar

reward. A set of new orders assigned him to Ft. McHenry in Baltimore. Although an officer in charge, Major Sprague, who paid the reward, probably considered Private Lynch just another deserter, no different from scores of others he had encountered, Lynch distinguished himself by eloping again shortly after his September apprehension and remained free until mid-December 1862. His skill in avoiding detection and arranging transportation was unbelievable. The officer of the guard, no doubt embarrassed by his miscalculation, immediately set out after his quarry, arresting him on the 14th of December in Albany.

This time, Private Lynch was transferred to Washington, D.C., where he remained a guest at the local jail. Eight months later, ingenuity carved another path to freedom. This cycle of arrest and escape continued for several more revolutions until Lynch's regiment finally contained him long enough to conduct a court-martial.

Perhaps the acrobatics of Private Lynch stirred a modicum of respect among some of his fellow soldiers. This man's determination epitomized strength, guile, and a reckless abandon for consequences. It had also cost the U.S. government a tidy sum. With each escape and subsequent apprehension, the reward for Lynch's capture had steadily risen, from an original measly five dollars to the princely sum of thirty dollars. The total amount of all rewards paid to apprehend Lynch exceeded ninety-two dollars.

Whatever roguish appeal Lynch might have commanded was apparently lost on the military officers of his court-martial. Multiple desertions were an insult to military authority and cried out for reprimand. The jury deliberated for a brief time before they demanded the ultimate penalty—the firing squad.

Lynch for once found that escape was impossible. With the only thing standing between him and a bullet being the executive approval of President Lincoln, Lynch made one last desperate gamble—he appealed for mercy.

Private Lynch drafted a carefully worded letter to President Lincoln. "I beg your Excellence to allow a few lines from the humblest of your subjects to find favor in your Sight." Private Lynch took a calculated risk. His strategy seemed to hinge on adopting a conciliatory tone without acknowledging any criminal responsibility. No apology was tendered, instead a direct petition was made: "[F]or my life I now plead and I trust in your clemency. I am a young man & in the full vigor of manhood & I do not wish to die." Private Lynch concluded his cautiously crafted appeal with a promise: "If my life be Saved it shall be devoted to whatever your Excellency may direct."

The power of the pen was indeed mighty. President Lincoln was apparently moved by compassion and issued Lynch a full pardon. The good fortune of Private Lynch continued. Following the executive order granting the pardon, Lynch was awarded an extended furlough, and he also laid claim to a three-hundred-dollar reenlistment bonus. The authorized thirty-day furlough period came and went. Inexplicably, Private Lynch deserted yet again.

Private Lynch's luck had finally run out. He was arrested near Buffalo in 1864 and returned for another judicial proceeding. His fate was certain: The verdict was guilty with the predictable sentence of death. No clemency could be expected now. The odyssey of Private Lynch ended with his execution.

A curious footnote added life to the saga of Private Lynch. About two weeks after his death, the Judge Advocate General sent a short note to the Headquarters Army of the Potomac. "Attention invited to omission from the record of prisoner's plea, in which the entire proceedings are invalidated . . . the Court can be recovered and the error, if mainly clerical, be corrected." Unfortunately for Private Lynch, any hope for a technical reprieve came too late. The response from Army Headquarters, perhaps seizing on the tendered explanation, endorsed "that the omission referred to was a *clerical* one."

As the pace of the Civil War accelerated, so did the number of executions in the Union Army. The years 1861 and 1862 jointly accounted for only a score of deaths, but there was a threefold increase the next year. The upward trend continued through 1864, when almost a hundred men were executed. The last full year of the war produced a minor downward drift. Even so, the number of executions in 1865 approached the century mark.[17]

The increasing pace of executions set in motion from 1863 was troubling. Many factors contributed to the relative popularity of the death sentence. Attitudes among many military officers hardened. A sagging support for the war, dragged down by the length of the conflict, undermined recruiting and retention. Those already bound to military service who deserted faced the prospect of severe punishment. The reality was different, since desertion was common but actually rarely punished. Public executions dramatized the risk of punishment but did little to deter it. One army unit was grimly determined to change this.

The Army of the Potomac sentenced fifty soldiers to death during a six-month campaign. Beginning in late November 1864, they conducted executions on a weekly basis.[18] Aggressive prosecutors presented to accommodating courts-martial, but despite the weekly spectacle, soldiers were not intimidated. As one observer from the time noted, "The wife of a man in my own company brought him a suit of citizen's clothing to desert in, which he availed himself of later; but citizen's clothes, even, were not always necessary to ensure safety for deserters."[19]

Some deserters vigorously resisted apprehension. These individuals generally had a good reason, as some were vicious criminals. Desertion was their least violent act. Once free of military control, they carried out serious assaults, murders, and rapes. According to the Records of the Adjutant General's office, Sgt. George McDonald of the 3rd Regiment, Maryland Volunteer Cavalry, was an example of this sort—one who vehemently fought both arrest and conviction. The prosecution charged Sergeant McDonald with desertion and two specifications of assault with intent to kill. Eight officers: two lieutenants, three captains, a major, one lieutenant colonel, and a full colonel, were assigned to Sergeant McDonald's general court-martial. A few days later, one of the three captains was removed, possibly a result of legal challenge.

Capt. A. G. Hennisee was appointed the judge advocate, and the case was tried in Baltimore, Maryland. Two weeks after convening the court-martial, the judge advocate went before the members explaining the delay. Captain Hennisee apologized for the inconvenience but acknowledged that assembling the witnesses was proving to be a difficult task, requiring yet a few more days for completion. The court reluctantly adjourned; however, the news was no better when the members reconvened. Several witnesses, including a key officer, were not immediately available. Ten more days would pass before all the players were in place and the legal proceedings could begin. The customary challenge of jury members was waived by the accused. Members then took an oath promising full and fair consideration of the facts to follow. The charges were read to Sergeant McDonald who, as usual, had no legal counsel.

The judge advocate charged that McDonald "had deserted the said Service, and was concealed in Montgomery County Maryland, at which place . . . did resist Sergeant Haugh and other soldiers . . . detailed and authorized to arrest him . . . that he the said McDonald . . . did discharge a loaded pistol and other deadly weapons at the said Sergeant and the other soldiers."

Sergeant McDonald listened quietly as the second specification of assault was lodged against him. This assault stemmed from a chance encounter between the accused and Ezekiel Moxley, a civilian. Their brief encounter near Clarksburg, Maryland, left Moxley injured.

The judge advocate accepted McDonald's plea of guilty to the desertion charge but not guilty to the other allegations.

The prosecution presented their case. Sgt. Jesse Haugh, a member of the Potomac Home Brigade, spoke first. He described Sergeant McDonald's arrest: Haugh and his squad of five men captured Sergeant McDonald near Laytonsville, a small city in the vicinity of Baltimore. As Sergeant Haugh approached the house where McDonald was hiding, his men quickly surrounded the building. McDonald was apparently alarmed and ran upstairs, leaving several of his friends downstairs. As Sergeant Haugh entered the home, McDonald's sympathizers doused the lights.

Angered, Sergeant Haugh "demanded them to get me a light— that if they did not I would put a light through some of them." His threat had little effect, so Haugh began looking for McDonald himself. As he began to ascend the steps the silence was punctured by the sound of a revolver cocking and the caged deserter saying, "I am ready for you." Haugh testified that he urged McDonald to surrender peaceably, but, uttering a violent oath, McDonald pledged his life before he would submit. Sergeant Haugh responded with a promise of his own: "I will smoke you out."

Sergeant Haugh was the right man for the job. Apparently possessed with dogged determination he was bound to overcome any resistance—and Sergeant McDonald was the obstacle. Haugh kept his word to make things hot as he set about "firing the bed." McDonald watched events unfold from the upper floor, but showed no signs that he meant to be captured. He fired a shot at Haugh, which sent forth a loud retort but no projectile.

Sergeant Haugh testified that he was fueled by anger, his brush with death being a galvanizing force. Haugh vividly recalled, "I then fired the house and he [McDonald] did not come to the window until the floor commenced falling that he was standing on. When I found he would not come down, I ordered the men to fire through the roof and through the gable ends of the house." Sergeant McDonald fired several ineffective shots in return. McDonald was in a precarious position; the house was burning down around him, and he was in a no-win predicament: He could either be arrested and face death later, or die now in the fire.

"He came to the window and begged for his life," Sergeant Haugh testified. Admitting that at the time he was still inflamed with anger, Sergeant Haugh said he had responded, "You have got to burn." McDonald's pleas for mercy escalated, and finally, satisfied that his prey had suffered sufficiently, Sergeant Haugh relented. Sergeant McDonald was forced to throw out his shotgun, assorted handguns, and knives, but his gratitude was short-lived. In words that would haunt him later, Sergeant McDonald bragged, "It was a lucky thing that [you] did not come upstairs." He then indicated that he was prepared to blow Haugh's "brains out."

Sergeant Haugh's testimony at trial was colorful, compelling, and condemning. When finished, Haugh awaited the counterattack. Once again, the two men faced each other, but McDonald, lacking the assistance of legal counsel, was poorly prepared to cross-examine a witness. No sparks would fly from this last confrontation between McDonald and Haugh. Not a single question was fired off.

Sergeant McDonald's court-martial bore many typical hallmarks. Only a few witnesses were called, and evidence presented by the prosecution remained essentially uncontested since the accused conducted his own defense. Officers assigned as members of the jury were often unfamiliar with military jurisprudence. The judge advocate had a similar naïveté. Only a rudimentary appellate system existed, and opportunities to review the facts and legal procedures used in a court-martial were limited to the whims of senior commanders or presidential clemency. On the other hand, Sergeant McDonald's trial differed in a few respects. It was uncharacteristically slow, and the accused, with the exception of not cross-examining Sergeant Haugh, directed an aggressive self-defense.

The court-martial of Sgt. George McDonald resumed after a short adjournment. To the consternation and dismay of the jury members important witnesses were again delayed. The judge advocate, no doubt expecting further rebuke, offered a peremptory explanation. A number of witnesses summoned to appear had countered by ignoring the order. The judge advocate lost all patience and vowed to compel witness compliance—through arrest. Reluctant civilian participants would not thwart the power of the court.

Judge Advocate Hennisee spoke with the 8th Army Corps provost marshal. As proof of prior efforts, Hennisee showed the president of the court-martial his most recent letter directing the witnesses' presence and assuring the president of their cooperation. Their failure to appear was an insufferable embarrassment. The judge advocate urged the provost marshal to use the power of his office to arrest the stubbornly resistant witnesses. The provost agreed. "I sent detective Taft to Monocacy on Saturday with a letter to General Tyler to furnish a squad of mounted men to arrest these witnesses. I have not heard from them yet although I expected them here this morning. I will notify you as soon as they arrive."

The second day of testimony started promptly at 10:00 A.M. A small group of unenthusiastic civilian witnesses were in attendance, their attempts to snub the court-martial having failed miserably.

Ezekiel Moxley was the first civilian to testify. Moxley was a gregarious, locally well-known horse trader. The twenty-six-year-old native of New Market, Maryland, supplied the U.S. government with prime livestock. Moxley made regular trips to Washington, D.C., plying his trade. One of these excursions was marked by a dramatic turn of events.

Returning early from business in Washington, Moxley had the unfortunate luck to encounter Sergeant McDonald. The horse trader had briefly stopped in Rockville, Maryland, a small town to the north of Washington, to have a meal before starting the final leg of his journey home. Moxley met a postman, and the pair became fast companions. Moxley testified that, although he enjoyed the slightly more circuitous route home, it turned out to be a fateful diversion.

The traveling pair arrived in Clarksburg, the mailman's destination, in the early afternoon. Even though he was many miles from home, Moxley knew many people in the surrounding towns. "When I got there some of my friends came out where I was," Moxley testified. They passed a few amiable moments together until their casual conversation was rudely interrupted by a stranger, who aggressively challenged Moxley. "This man came up and says, 'Do you belong to the Government Service?' 'No,' said I. Says he, 'Does that horse belong to the Government Service?' Says I, 'Are you a Detective?' Says he, 'you d--d dirty s-n of a b---h, I will give you Detective.'"

Moxley was surely surprised when Sergeant McDonald followed his violent epithet by pointing a revolver at his victim's chest. The intended target was confused and frightened. "I have never done anything for you to shoot me," Moxley remembered saying. Moxley clearly did not understand the desperate circumstances motivating the stranger's actions. McDonald wanted a horse; he needed the safety afforded by distance from his regiment. With his pistol aimed at the hapless civilian, Sergeant McDonald demanded Moxley climb down from his mount. The horse dealer begrudgingly complied, and, when McDonald directed him to back away from his horse, Moxley ruefully recalled, "I took it . . . just as orderly as a dog." "It is very hard for a man to have to take his hand off his own horse," Moxley complained to McDonald, who, at that point was a powder keg of nervous energy. Moxley's bitter comment apparently ignited the soldier, because, without warning, McDonald pulled the trigger.

Fortunately for Moxley, the bullet passed cleanly through his lower leg. Hobbled and humiliated, Moxley must have been further incensed by the lack of support from the other onlookers, as Sergeant McDonald coolly rode off with his horse. Before departing, McDonald quelled any thought of resistance from the group of thirty observers by pointing his handgun menacingly in their direction. The insult Moxley suffered that fateful day resurfaced a few weeks later at the court-martial. Moxley testified that it "was a pretty smart meeting there." There were "two constables and two magistrates. They could have taken him. They all appeared to be afraid of him."

Sergeant McDonald began the cross-examination. "Did you or not take me to be in my senses, when I shot?" he asked. Moxley retaliated, "you had sense enough to shoot me." Down but not out, McDonald tried a different approach, "Was I or not a sober man?" Moxley must have relished the chance to savage his assailant's defense. He completely sidestepped the question. "I never saw you before. I am very sorry I ever did see you. You have put me to a heap of trouble and misery I have suffered."

Moxley was a good witness for the prosecution, but the same could not be said of William Talbott, who had been instrumental in bringing the military to Sergeant McDonald's hideaway. Perhaps fearing retribution from McDonald's neighbors, Talbott appeared to be beset with a poor memory. His testimony was vague and proved nothing, and he was the prosecution's final witness.

In the typical court-martial, the jury heard evidence only from the prosecution, the defense being reduced to a simple supplication from the accused. Sergeant McDonald continued to defy expectations, by having two witnesses who would testify on his behalf. The first was Joseph Thompson, owner of the property where the drama had unfolded. Thompson first focused on the home's construction, particularly the cracks in the floor. McDonald's goal was to prove that the spaces between the floorboards were too narrow for him to have thrust a pistol through. Thompson's lack of pretrial preparation was exposed when his witness disagreed. Thompson conceded there were half-inch cracks in the floor, since it "was laid out in green planks and the plank had shrunk."

If Sergeant McDonald was embarrassed by his opening mistake, it caused only a momentary stumble. Quickly regaining the initiative, he challenged the accusation that he had fired a weapon. Here he made headway, as doubt was cast; Thompson, although possibly not within hearing range, could not verify the prosecution's claim that a pistol had been discharged. A different aspect of Thompson's testimony was more compelling. Thompson swore that the shotgun, allegedly fired during the fracas, was his. Thompson maintained that as a matter of practice, he always kept the shotgun unloaded—and none of his ammunition was missing. By this testimony, Sergeant McDonald hoped to prove that it was impossible for him to have fired the shotgun, thereby undermining Sergeant Haugh's credibility.

Thomas Warfield was the next defense witness. His trustworthiness was immediately in question, because he was a prisoner, confined for unstated crimes, alongside the accused. McDonald and his future witness had met each other in jail, and Warfield claimed to have been an eyewitness to the theft of Moxley's horse.

Sergeant McDonald asked only two questions of this witness. The first requested an account of the Moxley drama. "I come to the place [and] there was a great deal of excitement about it. I understand they said . . . when he [McDonald] shot . . . they did not suppose he shot to kill. Some thought it might have been an accidental shot. Moxley said, he did not think it was intended to kill him."

The second question Sergeant McDonald posed to his witness uncovered an important contradiction. "Did you or not hear Moxley say what he thought of me at the time?" Warfield recalled Moxley commenting at the time, "Well, you were very drunk."

Perhaps sensing some damage to the prosecution's case, the judge advocate launched a blistering cross-examination of Warfield. The jury members also probed the witness but no one was able to budge the unflappable Warfield. One court member pointedly asked, "Have you or not had an interview with the Accused since he has been confined?" Warfield retained his composure while denying having had any "Private interview" with McDonald. The last question put to this witness focused on his relationship with McDonald. Warfield remained resolute when probed about any jailhouse conversations. He did acknowledge that conversations occasionally took place between the two, but beyond that admission Warfield denied any insinuation linking the pair to a conspiracy. The court-martial ended with Warfield's testimony, and Col. G. A. Pierson, president of Sergeant McDonald's court-martial, retired with his fellow members to begin deliberations.

Sergeant McDonald was obviously a fighter. With little more than a rudimentary knowledge of military law, he nonetheless directly challenged the prosecution and assembled his own witnesses.

Time never favored most soldiers accused of a crime. War afforded little opportunity for in-depth pretrial criminal investigations or defense preparation. Courts-martial diverted precious manpower from the business of war. Deterrence was another reason courts-martial moved at such a quick pace. The military hoped that swift convictions would dissuade future malefactors. All these factors worked in tandem, tilting the scales of justice toward a successful prosecution, and these same factors loomed large in most military trials.

It was a somber procession that reassembled after a few hours of discussion. Two-thirds of the court members found, after "having maturely considered the evidence," that Sgt. George McDonald was guilty of two specifications of assault with intent to kill and one count of desertion. For these combined crimes McDonald was sentenced "to be shot to Death with musketry, at such time and place as the

Commanding General may direct." Sergeant McDonald's spirited defense had failed.[20]

According to the Records of the Adjutant General's office, the distasteful story of Sgt. Charles Sperry, 13th New York Cavalry, tolerated no such fuzzy comparisons. His sordid tale was distinctly different. Picket duty is boring, and drawing guard duty late at night is even worse. Sergeant Sperry was in charge of a small detail ordered to perform guard duty on a warm summer night in 1864, near Langley, Virginia. The idleness and tedium combined with the still night air to stimulate Sperry's mind and his attention apparently drifted toward daydreaming to break the monotony.

Cavalry soldiers enjoyed the freedom their military pursuits provided. As a mounted soldier Sergeant Sperry had some free reign to explore the local countryside. Searching for enemy troops, foraging, or scouting brought Sperry into intimate contact with the local population. During one of his assigned cavalry missions Sperry spied the Nelson home and the teenage girl who lived there.

Later that night, near midnight, Sperry shared his plan to return to the Nelson home with a few other members of his guard. Apparently bolstered by his comrades' support, Sergeant Sperry led the malevolent crew on horseback to the Nelson home. Somewhere along the route a quantity of liquor was obtained, and Sergeant Sperry fortified himself liberally.

The Nelson home was dark and quiet when the cavalry troop rode up. Confident that the ruse would succeed, the soldiers had agreed to use the pretext of searching for guerrillas to gain entry to the Nelson home. The soldiers shouted and pounded on the front door, and shortly, clad only in his nightdress, Mr. Nelson opened the door. Sergeant Sperry and his gang pounced on their stunned victim, and several of the men quickly subdued Mr. Nelson. Apparently dazed and confused by the sudden turn of events, Mr. Nelson submitted to his captors. The remaining cavalrymen, led by Sperry, quickly fanned out and systematically searched the house. Several young men who lodged in the Nelson home were hustled into a spare room, where another soldier silently but forcefully barred their exit.

So far the mission had unfolded like clockwork. Each man had assumed his role without much guidance. Sergeant Sperry meanwhile had obtained a lantern, and, by its feeble glow, undertook a search for the teenage girl. Running into each room of the Nelson home, Sergeant Sperry held the lantern up and illuminated the face of each family member. In his excitement, he never stopped to realize that the light illuminated his face as well.

Sperry found Annie, the teenage girl, in Mrs. Nelson's bedroom. Grabbing her viciously, he dragged the screaming fifteen-year-old into the adjacent bedroom in an attempt to force himself on her. Although her slight frame was no match against the burly soldier, she fought gamely. When Sperry forcibly sought to undress her, Annie fought back, leading Sperry to strike her on the head. Blood gushed from the wound, but Sperry continued his attack.

While Sperry was brutalizing Annie, Mrs. Nelson seized the opportunity to flee for help. After running nearly half a mile, Mrs. Nelson stumbled onto a small cavalry unit and begged them for help. The alarmed soldiers scooped up Mrs. Nelson and rode like the wind.

Sergeant Sperry was initially so preoccupied with the unexpectedly combative Annie that he did not hear the cavalry rescuers ride up. Almost too late, Sperry recognized his peril and fled the house. Fortunately, Annie, beaten and bruised, survived the lascivious attack undefiled. Sperry was apprehended a short distance from the Nelson home. His protests were brushed aside after several family members confirmed his role as the principal perpetrator. Their positive identification of him was aided by the light of Sergeant Sperry's own lantern, which had helped burn his image into their memories. Sperry was returned under guard to his regiment and charged with "quitting the guard without urgent necessity or leave, drunkenness on duty, assault and battery with intent to commit a rape."

The trial moved quickly. Sergeant Sperry's defense was limited; he acted as his own counsel. In remarks to the jury, Sergeant Sperry frankly admitted his unauthorized absence from the picket detail. Although it was dull duty, the security watch prevented surprise attacks, and dereliction of this responsibility was considered a grave offense. Sperry's drunkenness while on duty was "proved by abundant testimony." Neither of the foregoing accusations, however, assaulted the jury's sensibilities as much as the attempted rape charge did. This dissolute, depraved crime provoked a stern judgment. "The number of offenses against military and social law, which this ruffian is proved to have committed seems to call for the enforcement of the sentence to its fullest extent." His fate was sealed, and after a brief period of deliberation, the military jury expressed their opinion: Sergeant Sperry was guilty of capital offenses. The jury's moral repugnance was reflected in the sentence—death by musketry.

The court-martial record recounting Sperry's story captures the jury members' disgust, leaving little doubt as to the outcome. Although Sperry's guilt seemed evident based on the verbatim record, his lack of legal representation was a troubling footnote to this trial.[21]

Pvt. James Preble, a soldier of the 12th New York Volunteer Regiment, committed a similar, sordid crime. As it had with the Sperry case, alcohol played a prominent role in Preble's misdeeds.

Oliver Bedard's house was a comfortable abode for Souisa Bedard, Setitia Croft, and Rebecca Drake. Souisa was Mr. Bedard's seventeen-year-old daughter, Setitia Croft was an unmarried woman of fifty-eight, and Rebecca Drake was a twenty-three-year-old woman. Rebecca affectionately referred to Setitia as "Aunt Croft," and under her prudent guidance, the two younger women lived a simple life. In the Bedard household, she reigned as the undisputed matriarch. Aunt Setitia Croft had never married, and her romantic sentiments had never been openly expressed. Years of cloistered life had left its mark. Although slender and delicate, Setitia had not aged well; she looked much older than fifty-eight.

Private Preble discovered Bedard's house, and its female boarders, probably by accident. The young women apparently immediately struck his fancy, and his mind was likely flooded with base thoughts, which were only made worse by his consumption of alcohol.

Lieutenant Pierson wearily received the news that one of his troops was causing a ruckus at Oliver Bedard's house. The lieutenant directed Sgt. Arthur Nood to investigate the matter. Sergeant Nood took Pvt. James Hogan with him, and together the pair rode out to Bedard's house.

The Bedard home came into view just as Nood and Hogan crested a small rise. Preble's horse was hitched outside. Dismounting from his horse, Sergeant Nood walked to the front door and rapped loudly. A few seconds passed with no response. Nood was on the verge of knocking more forcefully when he heard a faint groan coming from inside. Sergeant Nood ran to the back door, hoping to find it open, but unfortunately it was securely locked. Alarmed and fearing the worst, Sergeant Nood assaulted the door with his shoulder; the entryway yielded to his weight.

The sight that met Nood would have been most unsettling. An elderly woman, covered with blood, came stumbling out of an adjoining room. Nood asked the woman if she had been shot, and in a quiet, quaking voice, Setitia Croft whispered, "no . . . I was raped." In response to Nood's momentary hesitation Setitia Croft pointed to the bedroom, where her assailant could be found.

Preble heard the commotion outside the bedroom, but apparently, he was not of a mind to move. When Sergeant Nood entered the room, Preble looked up and laughed, but Nood found no humor in the grotesque scene that confronted him. Private Preble was lying on his side, wearing an irksome expression. His pants were unbuttoned, soaked with blood, and limply hanging from his hand was a service revolver.

Sergeant Nood immediately snapped an order at Private Preble to get up, but Preble just ignored him and rolled over. Nood responded to this insolent behavior by pushing and dragging Preble outside. While Nood was preoccupied inside the house, his companion, Private Hogan, who was posted outside, was initially oblivious to the unfolding events.

In later testimony, Private Hogan admitted that he was daydreaming when Sergeant Nood and Private Preble came tumbling out of the house. "The first thing I saw was James Preble heaved out of the door with his Privates hanging out of his pants and his pants and shirt in that region all covered with blood. He had some liquor in him but was not so very drunk. As soon as he got out [of] the house he commenced laughing."

Preble was now outside the house and lying on the ground. The disgusted Sergeant Nood asked Hogan to get Preble on his horse. Private Hogan reached down to assist Preble to his feet but it proved to be an unnecessary gesture. Private Preble stumbled to his feet and mounted his horse. With an idiotic grin, Preble boasted, "that he had done more work than the whole battalion had that day." Hogan took that as a curious remark, and, only later, when Sergeant Nood filled in the details of the crime, did Preble's crass comment make sense.

Private Preble was accused of two specifications of assault with intent to commit rape and one charge of rape. Sergeant Nood, Private Hogan, and all three women were prepared to testify. The prosecutor carefully outlined the sordid facts. As the story unfolded, it became clear that the two younger women were Preble's real targets; only out of vindictive frustration had Setitia Croft been attacked.

Souisa Bedard, the youngest member of the house, was Preble's first victim. Surprised by the intruder's presence in their home, Souisa still managed to keep her wits. Preble, in a mildly drunken condition, rambled up to Souisa, and, putting his arm boldly around her, he signaled his intent. Muttering, "He'd be d_m'd if he wasn't a going to do just what he was a mind to with me." Souisa feared the worst. Any lingering doubts about Preble's motives were dispelled when he "pulled up his shirt exposing everything." Souisa testified that Private Preble vainly made an effort to throw her to the ground, but she managed to free herself and run outside. A few minutes later, with great trepidation, she returned inside. As she feared, Preble had cornered his next victim, Rebecca Drake. As Rebecca would testify, "He used all kinds of vulgar language. Such expressions as that he intended to have criminal connection with me or die. Exposed his person all that he could and walked around the house with pistol in his hand."

Rebecca Drake exhibited an astonishing composure. Hoping for a moment's distraction, she was rewarded with a lapse of attention from her assailant. She instantly fled the house, followed by Souisa, and together they hid among the fodder stacks. Preble pursued the two women but his frenzied search failed. At this juncture, it might have been wise for Private Preble to figure he was knee-deep in trouble and had been outflanked by two girls, but he would not leave unsatisfied.

Preble spotted Setitia Croft and demanded to know the whereabouts of the two missing women, but Setitia steadfastly refused to answer him. Private Preble pointed his revolver at Setitia, ordering her inside. She resisted, but was shoved inside the house, and with his gun cocked, Preble forced her into the bedroom. Setitia pled for mercy "but the more I begged the worse he acted and he threw me down on the bed and there gave me my ruin and he knows it too for he was not so drunk as he tried to make out."

Preble stifled any screaming by threatening to kill Setitia. She complied, and, following the twenty-minute ordeal, she dragged herself from the bedroom. Almost immediately upon her exit from the room, Sergeant Nood was upon the scene.

Even the best attorney would have difficulty defending such barbarism. Perhaps the sober and reflective Private Preble agreed. At his court-martial Preble offered no witnesses, evidence, or even the typical plea for mercy. The court-martial verdict seemed automatic. Private Preble was guilty and would face the firing squad.[22]

Pvt. Michael Wert, Company G, 184th Pennsylvania Volunteers, was a simpleminded youth. Whether it was from patriotic fervor or from a peer's suggestion, Michael Wert joined the military. Eight months later Private Wert was no longer fighting for his country but for his own life. This battle was not part of any southern campaign but instead was fought as part of a political-legal crusade to stem losses suffered through desertion. The weapons deployed were not rifles and cannons, they were words, but the reality of death was just as real from either weapon. Wert had received no training to defend himself against these instruments of destruction. Skilled attorneys were expensive, leaving Private Wert no option but to proceed alone. With scarcely any preparation, Wert entered the courtroom gamely self-assured but facing a formidable challenge.

Private Wert was arraigned on a single charge of desertion. The judge advocate was prepared to show that Wert had deserted while on picket guard "after having been duly posted, did, willfully leave his post, with the intention of deserting to the enemy." Not a shadow of doubt flickered across Wert's face when the accusation was made. His implacable confidence drew strength from the numerous reassurances he had received. His friends, now defense witnesses, would surely explain the whole mess away. Wert was probably convinced that once the members of the court-martial heard his story as told by his character references, his innocence would be established. Unwitting and gullible, this simpleminded soldier listened quietly to the parade of prosecution witnesses.

Capt. Francis F. Reynolds of the 59th Regiment, New York Volunteers, was the first prosecution witness. Captain Reynolds was the commanding officer assigned to monitor picket details. His testimony began with a general description of the shape and position of the picket line that stretched in front of Fort Conahey, Petersburg, Virginia. "It was a curved line. The posts on the left were thrown back to the Squirrel Level Road. The right post was in front of the road." Captain Reynolds remembered the area as "woody" and the weather as cold and rainy. The only extraordinary event Captain Reynolds testified about was the capture of Private Wert. When questioned at the time by his commanding officer, Wert had sheepishly acknowledged abandoning his picket. Captain Reynolds pressed for more, and in response, Private Wert broadened his disclosures.

Captain Reynolds continued his testimony. Private Wert had dropped his accoutrements before leaving picket post number nine. He was later apprehended at post number sixteen. At this point in Captain Reynolds's narration, Private Wert interrupted. This was his first opportunity to cross-examine the witness. He did so by asking two questions that bore on the point of capture and the distance he allegedly traveled. Private Wert recognized the incriminating nature of those admissions and wisely sought to challenge them.

Under Private Wert's cross-examination Captain Reynolds guessed that pickets nine and sixteen were separated by a distance of about 1,600 feet. Vedettes were replaced every two hours. These mounted sentries were assigned specific posts, and it seemed plausible that

Private Wert could have easily negotiated the 1,600 feet during the sentry's absence.

Lt. James McGowan, testifying for the prosecution, was the first to hint at some unusual behavior. McGowan recalled the early morning arrest of Wert near picket sixteen. Lieutenant McGowan was surprised to see the errant soldier. Naturally suspicious, he briefly interrogated Wert. "I asked him his name, and Regiment and where he belonged, and what he was doing." Private Wert's response was curious, "the Yanks were going to make a charge in the morning . . . they were going to make a charge on the left." The remark was either a clever contrivance or the rambling of a confused individual.

The prosecution witness offering the most information was Sgt. William Fitzgerald. Sergeant Fitzgerald was in command of picket posts six, nine, and eleven. In his testimony, Fitzgerald recalled Wert being alert and energetic. Private Wert's first turn at picket duty began near midnight. As the shifts were exchanging personnel two hours later, an unusual event intervened. While being relieved, Wert made an offer to stand vedette post for two additional hours. It was an odd request. Sergeant Fitzgerald's initial impulse was to refuse the offer. His principal concern centered on taking a man out of turn, but for some unexplained reason, the sergeant's resistance faded. Perhaps, it was partly due to Private Wert's insistence. Sergeant Fitzgerald testified, "I finally posted him at the vedette post, it was 2 o'clock A.M."

About ninety minutes after accepting Private Wert's proposal, Sergeant Fitzgerald made his routine inspection rounds. He silently noted that Wert was battle ready with his knapsack, canteen, and haversack properly secured. Sergeant Fitzgerald continued on his way, reassured by the pickets' vigilance. Another fifteen minutes passed. The ritual of rotating the troops was again set in motion. Sergeant Fitzgerald and the designated relief, traveling separately, arrived at Private Wert's vedette post almost simultaneously at four o'clock. Both were surprised to find the posted sentry gone and the ground littered with a rifle, cartridges, and a belt.

Sgt. T. D. Phillips, another prosecution witness, was responsible for posts fifteen and sixteen. Phillips testified that that night's boredom was punctuated by a most unusual incident. A soldier riding down the dark road dimly came into view. He stopped abruptly in front of the posted sentry. "Good evening boys," was the stranger's cheery introduction. Sergeant Phillips politely exchanged social greetings, but remained at a loss to explain his visitor's presence. Driven by curiosity and military necessity, the sergeant probed his caller. Wert simply replied, "I am lost," but the cynical sergeant thought otherwise. "I think you are not lost, I think you are all right, you are with the Johnny's now."

Amazingly, Private Wert assumed he had stumbled into the midst of the rebel force. With no additional prompting, he disclosed Yankee positions and strategies. "The Yanks are going to make a charge on you in the morning, either here, or the left." Perhaps it was the dim light that confused him, but soon it apparently dawned on Wert that something was amiss. "You have Yank clothing on," the puzzled Wert observed. The sergeant, eager to encourage more incriminating statements, kindled the deception. By alluding to a recent victorious skirmish against the Yanks, the sergeant set the trap. "We got their clothing and give them a pretty good thrashing." The ruse continued a few moments longer. Finally, satisfied that Private Wert was a traitorous deserter, Sergeant Phillips sprang the trap. The trap set by Phillips was tight. It closed even more during the court-martial, and the prosecution phase of the trial ended with his dramatic testimony.

Private Wert seemed oblivious to his peril, and he continued a vain struggle. He presented one witness, Lt. William Bell, his company commander, to speak on his behalf. Bell provided a sympathetic portrait.

"What has been my character as a soldier?" Private Wert asked of his commander, to which Lieutenant Bell responded favorably. There were many occasions, the lieutenant insisted, when Private Wert could have deserted, but he never did. In Bell's opinion Wert was a trusted soldier, and Lieutenant Bell was impressed with his young charge's bravery under fire. It was a strong endorsement, but from this point forward the lieutenant wandered into less flattering territory.

Possibly this jaunt was geared toward extricating Private Wert from the trap set by Sergeant Phillips. "I am almost certain that he is very weak minded. He is very easily controlled, and would believe almost anything a man would tell him, who got his confidence. He has scarcely judgment enough to know right from wrong." The testimony implied that Sergeant Phillips had tricked a "confession" from a feebleminded soldier guilty only of being lost.

Lieutenant Bell's testimony was valuable, coming from an officer who had been familiar with the accused for the past eight months. Unfortunately, Private Wert lacked the sophistication and resources to exploit this advantage. The question raised regarding the accused's mental capacity was never answered. No physician examined Private Wert. Family members did not testify. Closing arguments by the accused were weak.

The military court recessed and pondered the evidence. A short while later, the presiding officer intoned, "having maturely considered the evidence adduced, [we] find the accused Private William Wert . . ." guilty. Private Wert was executed by a firing squad. Wert's defense failed to strike any sympathetic cords. The condition of his mental state, succinctly portrayed by his unit commander, apparently resonated with no one.[23]

At least, in that respect, Pvt. Henry Hamilton, Company D, of the United States Colored Infantry, was more successful. While still succumbing to the same fate as Private Wert, Hamilton's pleadings were more effective, perhaps in part due to the skills of Lt. O. A. Carpenter, who served as Hamilton's defense counsel.

Pvt. Henry Hamilton faced three charges: "joining in a mutiny, offering violence against his superior officer, and disobedience of orders." The charges grew out of a riot that engulfed the company in December 1863 at Ship Island, Mississippi. Tensions had been smoldering in the unit for weeks. A number of gripes, such as slow pay, smug insubordination, and racial prejudice, were held in check through military discipline. The pent-up discord finally vented itself.

Captain Barthoff had ordered the arrest of Pvt. Henry Cornish. In response, Private Cornish reluctantly walked toward the guardhouse, while several men who were milling about silently observed the incident unfold.

The arrest of Pvt. Henry Cornish sparked murmured protest among his fellow soldiers. Like a magnet attracting metal filings, soldiers were slowly drawn to Cornish. Pvt. Murray Hamilton, later called as a defense witness, saw the trouble brewing. "When they came for Cornish to take him to the guard-house, and the men began to cry out that they should not take him there, I knew there was going to be trouble. I went away when the disturbance broke out, to another company street."

Pvt. Murray Hamilton's disappearance was hardly noticed. There were almost 300 men in various stages of supporting the uprising. Those closest to Cornish were the most vocal rioters. Among them was Pvt. Henry Hamilton who was close enough to almost touch Cornish.

Lt. Edward Peas was the officer of the day. The developing disturbance demanded action. Making his way quickly to the center of the fracas, Lieutenant Peas observed a group of roughly 200 men surrounding the hapless sergeant who was nudging Cornish into the guardhouse. Two men were holding rifles, in a blatant attempt to thwart the detention of Cornish. Only decisive action could quell the bubbling discontent. Without evincing any outward fear, Lieutenant Peas strode into the midst of the malcontents, his attention focused on the two armed rioters. Turning toward Hamilton, the determined lieutenant ordered him back to quarters. In response, Hamilton pointed a bayonet at the officer of the day.

Peas was not intimidated by the show of force. Grabbing the shank of the bayonet, Peas attempted to arrest Hamilton, but his effort was in vain. A tense but brief stalemate followed until Peas beat a hasty retreat. His actions may have looked like a victory to the rioters, but their interpretation was in error, as Peas immediately relayed the threat to Col. Albert A. Fellows. Returning with Lieutenant Peas to the company street, Colonel Fellows was temporarily successful in arresting a suspected ringleader. Peas meanwhile tried to regain control over Henry Cornish as a flurry of rocks was hurled in protest. The combined efforts of several officers finally restored military control.

Private Hamilton's court-martial transcripts scarcely suggested a motive for the mass disintegration of military authority. The rest of the record documented the accused's defense. The typical parade of prosecution witnesses described the mutiny. Even with the assistance of an attorney, the defense was weak. Just prior to jury deliberations, Hamilton exercised his privilege to make a closing statement, and the court granted a brief recess for Hamilton to prepare his statement.

"I was out in my company street, cleaning my gun when the guard came after Cornish, and the way I happened to have my bayonet fixed—there were four or five together in the tent, and all the way I could tell mine was by fixing it. I did not intend to hurt anyone. I went to my quarters when the officer of the day ordered me to. I can't read or write, and I beg the mercy of the court on account of my ignorance."

Mutiny was a severe breech of military law. Usurping military authority violates the most basic concept of an army. The court-martial members surely endorsed that notion. As a consequence, Pvt. Henry Hamilton's conviction was certain. His crime also justified the death penalty—or so the requisite two-third majority concluded. In an extraordinary move, two jury members protested the harsh sentence. Their concerns were submitted in writing as an "Appendix A" to the official court-martial record:

"We the undersigned, members of a General Court-martial . . . recommend, to executive clemency Henry Hamilton. . . . We do this on account of his manifest ignorance and in consideration that—while his criminality was far from being the highest in degree of its kind, the extreme measure of punishment was affixed there to by the sentence of the court." Two captains, including the court-martial's judge advocate, supported leniency. Both were overruled.[24]

The last hope for clemency was vested in presidential authority. There were no rules, save conscience, that guided these momentous decisions, in which two competing philosophies clashed. Appeals for mercy were countered by arguments demanding punishment as a general deterrent.

"I don't believe it will make a man any better to shoot him," President Lincoln said, expressing his philosophy on executions. Lincoln's experience as an attorney, politician, humanitarian, and wartime president uniquely positioned him to fairly review courts-martial death sentences. Somewhere sandwiched between governing the Union and fending off political enemies, Lincoln expended enormous resources reviewing numerous death sentences.[25]

During the war several hundred thousand soldiers deserted, and perhaps a third of them were arrested. Despite this dismal record, more men were executed for desertion than for any other crime. President Lincoln probably understood that the death penalty had no practical effect on desertion rates. Paradoxically, the inequitable dispensation of justice may have fostered losses by encouraging a sense of unfairness.

Another potential flash point for military injustice occurred when martial law was imposed to control occupied Southern cities. It was political insanity to breed resentment through unduly harsh military law. Military arrest for civilian transgressions, depending on the nature of the offense, ensnared the unwitting perpetrator in a web of military authority. Conducting a military trial prevented southern sympathies from infecting a jury, as they might have if jurors were drawn from the civilian population. The story of Dr. David Minton Wright unfolded against such a backdrop.[26]

Norfolk, Virginia, fell to Union control early in the war. The terms of surrender were arranged between the town council members and Gen. John Ellis Wool, Commander of the Union forces. During the brief period of General Wool's administration mutual respect prevailed.

Gen. Benjamin Butler was appointed as the next commander following Wool's departure, and conditions in the city soured rapidly. Private belongings were routinely seized and mysteriously vanished. A smothering repression crept over the citizenry. The ultimate humiliation that fired local passions occurred "when General Butler sent over Negro troops who took possession of the sidewalks and rudely thrust both ladies and gentleman from their way." The trial that captivated the city was born from this seemingly innocuous act that occurred in 1862.

Two dissimilar stories emerged. Dr. Wright and his civilian witnesses agreed on one version. Their sympathetic account portrayed Dr. Wright as a champion lashing out at oppressors. It played well with the locals, but they were not sitting in judgment. Dr. Wright, acting impulsively and imprudently, gave voice to a collective frustration. Most citizens, forced from the sidewalk by the Union troops, suffered this indignation quietly, but Dr. Wright was unable to hold his tongue. Jostled off the pedestrian path, the angry physician cried, "How dastardly." The exclamation reached the ears of the troop commander, Lt. A. A. Sanborn. Perhaps on guard for insurrection, Lieutenant Sanborn wheeled suddenly and drew his sword. Dr. Wright never traveled with a firearm, but an unknown witness to the evolving drama forced a pistol into his hand.

Now armed, Dr. Wright ordered the lieutenant back, but the officer ignored the injunction and advanced. A shot, fired from the doctor's pistol, smashed into the officer's hand. The wounded officer rashly commanded his troops to arrest his antagonist. All the while, the lieutenant continued threatening Dr. Wright, who in response fired again. Bleeding from a mortal wound, the determined officer grappled with Wright. It was to be the lieutenant's last battle. Almost immediately following the lieutenant's death, a provost arrested Dr. Wright.

The military's goal during the trial was to oppose Wright's chivalrous defense of southern virtues. Military authorities painted a malevolent picture. According to the prosecution, Dr. Wright was waiting at a store, and let loose a volley of oaths as the parade of troops passed by. The military maintained that Wright carried a concealed weapon, which he fired twice as Lieutenant Sanborn turned to order his arrest. The two shots struck Sanborn, and a brief struggle between the two consumed the officer's remaining energy. He died in the store.

Dr. Wright was not without means, and hired capable attorneys.

His initial team, provoked by the court-martial procedures, retired in protest. The court had refused to accept Dr. Wright's proffered plea of insanity. The trial, mired in controversy, began on that inauspicious note. Throughout the trial, Dr. Wright excited the pity of his family and friends. He was denied a civilian trial and the plea of his choice. In addition, he suffered the public indignation of shuffling about in chains. Whenever transported to court, Wright attracted a sympathetic group of well-wishers. The desperate plight of the prisoner motivated at least one person.

Jail officials supported a liberal visitation policy. Each night close family members met with Dr. Wright; however, one night, the routine was noticeably altered. Miss Penelope, Wright's loyal daughter, driven by her father's humiliation, hatched a novel plan that she immediately set in motion. Arriving by herself that night, she silently entered her father's cell. Hushed voices and a snuffed candle drew the attention of the military guard, and an extra sentry was posted nearer the doctor's cell. Whatever mysteries unfolded in the dark went undetected by the sentry. After a few moments, Miss Penelope made known her desire to leave, and the sentry obligingly opened the door. The woman emerged, and, taking long, cautious strides, she left the guardhouse.

Seconds later, an excited guard apprehended the woman. His suspicions had been aroused by a chance observation—Miss Penelope seemed to have grown a bit during the time she had spent in the cell with her father. The guard cried out the alarm after confirming his suspicions. "Miss Penelope" turned out to be Dr. Wright ingeniously clad in female attire. Miss Penelope was discovered in the doctor's recently vacated bed. The part she was to play in the ruse was to lie quietly covered in the bed, with only her father's boots exposed. Neither Dr. Wright nor Miss Penelope was flustered or apologetic upon their discovery, although they surely regretted it.

Dr. Wright's court-martial "was immediately held; no extenuating circumstances were admitted, and the simple fact that an officer of the army had been slain by a rebel sympathizer outweighed all other considerations." Dr. Wright was found guilty of murder and promptly received the death penalty.

The death sentence had barely been pronounced, when forces loyal to the doctor rallied. There were no spontaneous or orchestrated street demonstrations. Instead, protest was organized around a letter-writing campaign. A similar theme was mentioned in each letter—Dr. Wright was a peculiar, idiosyncratic individual, with some no doubt commenting on his forgetfulness and dysphoria. Numerous testimonials strongly hinting that Dr. Wright was not of sound mind were delivered to President Lincoln.

President Lincoln must have been impressed with Dr. Wright's appeal for clemency. The pile of affidavits proclaiming Wright's insanity could not be easily dismissed; they were just too prodigious in number. Since the court-martial had imperiously dismissed any discussion of Dr. Wright's mental state, President Lincoln perhaps felt compelled to order an inquiry. It was the only equitable response to the court-martial's arrogance.

The commission, under the supervision of Dr. John P. Gray, was charged with taking, "in writing all evidence which may be offered on behalf of Dr. Wright. . . . All said evidence to be directed to the question of Dr. Wright's sanity. . . . When the taking of evidence shall be closed, you will report the same to me, together with your own conclusions as to Dr. Wright's sanity, both at the time of the homicide and the time of your examination. If you deem it proper, you will examine Dr. Wright personally, and you may, in your discretion, require him to be present, during the whole or any part of the taking of evidence."

Dr. Gray proceeded to Fort Monroe, Virginia, where Dr. Wright was jailed. With respect, deference, and quiet authority, Dr. Gray began his inquiry. Attorneys representing Dr. Wright were contacted, and after a short discussion, all parties agreed that Wright should be interviewed.

The inquiry into the mental state of Dr. Wright resembled a trial. Skillful defense attorneys represented the physician. It was the avowed purpose of the government judge advocate to prove Dr.

Wright sane. Both sides called thirteen witnesses to advance their position. While the attorneys were ensconced in witness selection and case preparation, Dr. Gray interviewed the accused.[27]

Dr. Wright impressed his colleague. He was a stately man who exuded a solemn tone. His long gray hair, impeccably manicured beard, quiet gaze, and philosophical eloquence ensured a measure of respect. Dr. Gray was not disappointed by this initial impression. Both physicians took a seat in the cramped jail quarters, and Dr. Wright waited patiently as Dr. Gray explained the purpose of their meeting. Sensitive to legal procedures, Gray offered to conduct the evaluation with defense counsel present, but Wright refused the offer.

The awkward anxiety of one physician examining the other was partially bridged through an exchange of social pleasantries. Both gave an account of their current professional duties, prior training, and interests. Throughout this exchange Dr. Gray was quietly assessing the competence of his colleague.

Dr. Wright proved himself to be a conscientious physician. In the course of contacts with local physicians and through scientific study, Wright stayed abreast of medical developments. That was an important ethical discovery that indicated Dr. Wright took the health of his patients seriously.

Dr. Wright had received his medical training at the University of Pennsylvania. He was a studious individual who was further distinguished as a peaceful man throughout his life. He was neither intemperate nor impatient, qualities he had cultivated through a lifelong commitment to his personal health. Following a careful diet and keeping regular hours were enduring practices. As he grew older, aged fifty-four in 1862, Dr. Wright was bedeviled by forgetfulness. The loss was gradual, and a daily calendar of duties prevented most lapses. His wife noted the problem and responded by politely reminding her husband each night of important appointments. A similar obliviousness crept into the physician's prescription writing routine. To prevent a grievous error, Dr. Wright adopted a regular practice of checking each medication prescription twice. By employing his own mnemonics and relying on his wife's gentle reminders, Dr. Wright avoided serious medical consequences. Dr. Gray probably made a mental note of this cognitive decline.

Dr. Gray adroitly turned the inquiry toward politics. The accused confirmed his predictable Southern sympathies, which unquestionably seasoned his political thoughts. By means of this overture, Gray was able to extend the discussion to the crime. Dr. Wright's recollection of events regarding the murder was similar to that of the prosecution. Following the shooting, a flood of contradictory thoughts had engulfed his mind. His first impulse had been to render medical assistance to the injured Lieutenant Sanborn, but the officer was beyond helping. The enormity of the deed overwhelmed Dr. Wright. Tears of grief, shame, and guilt could not wash away the consequences. Dr. Wright, a man dedicated to preserving life, had taken one. Several days of mental anguish finally yielded to a peaceful acceptance. Following the painfully honest description of his life and moral failures, Wright pointedly asked Gray his opinion, but the latter remained noncommittal.

Dr. Gray was reticent to make a frank admission. In his estimation, the medical interview with Dr. Wright had produced little evidence of mental illness. There was, for example, a complete lack of idiosyncratic, delusional thinking. The murder appeared to be the product of spontaneously inflamed passions, however; Dr. Wright's forgetfulness and lifelong dysphoria were troubling and deserved further attention. Witnesses called before the commission would settle that issue.

Both the defense and prosecution called thirteen witnesses. Curiously absent from the defense lineup were any members of Wright's family. Those who testified about Dr. Wright's behavior were mostly casual acquaintances, with a few notable exceptions.

G. W. Camp had known Dr. Wright for many years. His testimony for the defense was not helpful. Mr. Camp assured the commission, based on a close relationship, that Wright was of sound mind. It appeared to be a tactical error on the part of the defense to include this witness.

A more constructive witness, John D. Ghiselin, described Dr. Wright's depression. Just two days before the murder, Dr. Wright had received a great shock: The Confederate Army had suffered an important defeat at the obscure little town of Gettysburg, Pennsylvania. Among the many soldiers engaged in that battle was Dr. Wright's son. There were rumors of many casualties, and obtaining accurate news reports was agonizingly slow. The uncertainty about his son's fate tormented the father deeply. The defense witness, in describing Wright's turmoil, used terms such as *great depression* and *incoherence.*

The last important defense witness was Dr. Robert B. Turnstall, a local colleague. Dr. Turnstall provided ambiguous, contradictory observations. He noted "fits of despondency" and "eccentricities of manner" in Dr. Wright; however, the onset and severity of these symptoms was impossible to elicit from this witness.

The one remaining question involved the defendant's memory. Dr. Gray explored this subject with Dr. Turnstall. As he was with the preceding testimony, Gray was dissatisfied with Dr. Turnstall's account. The latter simply labeled Wright's prescriptions as odd, apparently based on little more than Turnstall's conclusion that Wright was an "independent character" who rarely consulted colleagues. In the interests of thoroughness, Gray reviewed Wright's prescriptions and concluded that, although they occasionally deviated from accepted practice, the prescriptions "exhibited no indications of insane caprice."

The prosecution witnesses were more persuasive. There was little deviation in their testimony. One after another, they exposed no peculiarities about the accused. The testimony of Charles A. Santos, a local chemist familiar with Wright's prescribing habits, was given great weight by Dr. Gray. The witness acknowledged oddities about Dr. Wright's medication orders, but that friendly admission was immediately diluted. According to the chemist's recollection, Dr. Wright's behavior was predictable and had remained unchanged for years.

Dr. Gray authored a lengthy report to President Lincoln at the conclusion of the commission. The opinion noted, "In Dr. Wright's own statements . . . he said that he committed the deed under an uncontrollable impulse. It has been impossible for me to arrive at the conclusion that this impulse was an insane one. . . . Dr. Wright was not suffering from delusion. . . . He was under the influence of a burst of passion." Dr. Gray dismissed the depression immediately preceding the murder and its cause. The roiling mental effects resulting from his son's possible death were not stretched far enough to justify Dr. Wright's extraordinary departure from his normally serene life.

An emotional news account described Dr. Wright's final day. "The day of execution had come, dark clouds obscured the heavens. . . . On reaching the street he [Dr. Wright] asked permission to look into his coffin . . . and he stood for some minutes and looked fondly at the daguerreotypes of his wife and children . . . hung up around the inside of his coffin. . . . He took leave of his clerical friends . . . knelt down . . . and then his soul returned to the God who gave it . . . and thousands followed his remains to their last resting place."[28]

A just legal system is fair. Crimes are carefully cataloged offenses that assault the social mores. Punishment is decided only after balancing the effects of retribution versus rehabilitation. Sometimes an imbalance occurs and a sense of inequity creeps in and the perpetrator's misconduct is blurred by sympathy. Some behaviors, while violating an established law, are imbued with a sense of nobility. Such was the ambiguous reception awaiting conscientious objectors.

Subscription to a pacifist religious doctrine was abruptly challenged by the war. Their vocal opposition to armed conflict exposed a small army of previously invisible pacifists. In many cases, the official response to the opposition was silence. By not elevating the discord, public debate could be limited and difficult national choices could be avoided. The problem was not eliminated; it was just displaced.

In some cases, sparks of religious discontentment set passions ablaze at the regimental level, with predictable consequences. Commanders had only a limited repertoire of interventions to wield in response to any defiant behavior.

There were no exceptions from the military draft countenanced on religious grounds. For the vast majority of religious men, this stirred no inner turmoil, but among members of some religious sects, such as the Quakers or Mennonites, a deep-seated aversion to war translated into draft opposition. The lack of a national policy recognizing conscientious objectors ensured a bumbling approach when the situation arose.

Pvt. Henry D. Swift was a pacifist. When his draft notice compelled military service he consented under duress. Swift was a member of the Religious Society of Friends, more generally known as Quakers. His belief system was decidedly antiwar. Private Swift reluctantly traveled from his South Dedham, Massachusetts, home to join the military, and, almost immediately upon arrival, he began a campaign of passive resistance. Swift stalwartly refused to participate in any military activity. From the military perspective, such defiance was intolerable and illegal, and Swift suffered accordingly.

Private Swift's first assignment was to the guardhouse. There he languished until a transfer to Long Island changed the scenery. Nothing else changed, including Swift's unbending defiance. A contest of wills followed. His commanding officers instituted punishment, but bucking and gagging had no effect on Swift's position. Other physical inducements were similarly ineffective. This stalemate could not continue, and Private Swift was bound to lose the struggle with his superior officers. He was court-martialed for his unrelenting insubordination. The death penalty assigned was sorely out of proportion with the offense.

The inequity of the sentence shook the Massachusetts congregation that called Private Swift a member. They rallied to his defense and petitioned the President. President Lincoln was swayed, and he issued an executive pardon, sparing Swift's life. It was a convoluted, dangerous path that Swift was forced to travel, to maintain his faith.[29]

Death penalty cases put both an accused soldier and military justice on trial. These serious legal cases unfolded against a larger and deadlier struggle that a divided nation was waging. Civil War court-martial practice was imperfect; too few defendants benefited by legal representation, and imposition of the death penalty should only have followed a unanimous jury verdict. In addition, the appellate system was weak in practice and relied heavily on the whims of senior authorities. Fortunately, compassion was frequently extended, often following a determined campaign by friends and family.

The focus of a divided America was squarely centered on waging battles and vilifying the enemy. Strict adherence to cumbersome legal procedure too often was seen as undermining the primary struggle. In a similar fashion, the imperative need to build a comprehensive medical service was initially neglected. As the war dragged on, with no end in sight, the early euphoria of quick victory faded. This sober realization forced a reconsideration of the proper role of both the legal and medical professions. Changes were more visible with medical care as that infrastructure steadily grew. Legal lessons were also learned. Each court-martial left an indelible record, sketched on paper, on the participants' minds, or both. Justice is perceived in this manner, and in a country governed by fairness, change is inevitable. Modern military law corrected many inequities that were so obvious during the Civil War; assignment of a defense counsel for every accused soldier became the norm, and designating that the death penalty required a unanimous vote of the jury. An automatic appeals process was put in place that guarantees an impartial review of the harshest sentences.

CHAPTER THREE

ALCOHOL AND THE LAW

"The sale or giving away of intoxicating liquor, wine, beer or cider is strictly prohibited . . . to all enlisted men . . . in this town."[1] Commanders surely understood alcohol-related misconduct. Orders forbidding the purchase or sale of spirits were common. Such resolve paradoxically coexisted with a benign attitude promoting the beverage. Troops were often rewarded by a free, command-sponsored indulgence. Alcohol was a common medicinal agent, which further served to blur sharp moral attitudes concerning its use. Perhaps not surprisingly, officers who imbibed excessively could expect a more lenient reaction than that afforded enlisted men.

Habitual drunkenness was considered by many in the Victorian era to be a moral defect; however, theories embracing an enlightened medical cause of alcohol disorders were beginning to emerge. Conflicting social perceptions swirled around alcohol: It was believed to be a therapeutic agent, a reward, a soporific to soften the hard edge of war, yet also the source of all evil behavior and moral decline. These conflicting notions about alcohol reverberated, and frequently collided, in the nineteenth-century practice of medicine, military law, and command. This ambiguity often bred inconsistent treatment of alcohol-related criminal behavior. It might be excused through commiseration or alternatively denounced as a moral depravity demanding public shaming. Serious misbehavior might justify incarceration. In these instances, alcohol served to amplify the call for punishment. Doctors prescribed alcohol, since its well-known anesthetic properties served as a numbing agent for many soldiers facing surgery. Commanders jealously guarded alcohol rations; it was a favorite means to motivate dispirited troops. Because of these overlapping attitudes, soldiers could easily cross an ill-defined line marking a transition to inappropriate alcohol use. When this occurred in the military a court-martial was assembled to pass judgment.

Col. William Weer was the commander of the military prison in Alton, Illinois, in 1864.[2] Life at any prison is never easy for the inmates or officers, but circumstances at Alton were extreme. The post commander was unpredictable, causing normal anxieties to be magnified. Commanders generally enjoyed a respect that accompanied their responsible positions. Most leaders used that respect wisely; they implicitly understood that men would more willingly follow a trusted leader. However, some military officers squandered that high esteem that was granted to them. Goodwill was dissipated through intimidation, abuse of authority, lack of knowledge, and inequity.

Colonel Weer exceeded any behavioral discretion allowed his office. His erratic conduct flowed from the bottle. Weer's staff initially excused the post commander's actions. A common rationalization minimized the obvious: The commander drank too much. Eventually, Colonel Weer's conduct escalated to a point that it threatened the safety of the prison. His heavy drinking was embarrassing, and there were an ever-increasing number of social gaffes. At the beginning of Colonel Weer's command, these had been isolated events, exclusively confined outside duty hours, but eventually his work was increasingly threatened by his use of alcohol.

Major Stephens worked closely with Colonel Weer and had grown increasingly concerned about his commander's decline. He pondered his options: Remain silent and supportive, or confront his commander's behavior. Neither was an attractive choice. For Major Stephens, deciding what course of action to pursue against his commander offered enormously risky choices. Perhaps it was inevitable that the ambivalence Major Stephens grappled with would be telegraphed to his commanding officer. Somehow, Colonel Weer must have read Major Stephen's internal doubts, generating suspicions about his subordinate's loyalty. The pretense for Colonel Weer to take action against a supposedly insubordinate junior officer no doubt sprang from an alcohol-influenced overreaction. In any event, Colonel Weer felt sufficiently threatened by Major Stephens to have him arrested by a small contingent of soldiers. Following his apprehension, the officer was hurried along back to the post. This seemingly senseless turn of events defied his understanding. Major Stephens's anxiety probably spiked as he entered the post under guard. The embarrassment was probably insufferable. The ignominious arrest was further aggravated by the fact that he would be confined in the guardhouse. As the door closed behind him, Major Stephens had only moments to consider his fate, as soon thereafter, an enraged Colonel Weer barged into the guardhouse. Glaring viciously at the prisoner, he lost all restraint. Physically striking the major, Colonel Weer vented, "Damn you, you are nothing but an impostor and a spy." The bewildered major could scarcely contain his anger and resentment.[3]

Conditions in the military hospital at Alton had steadily deteriorated throughout the course of Colonel Weer's command. Staff and patients were united in their criticism, and blame was squarely placed on the post commander. Those affected complained that Weer "was so drunk as to be unfit for duty; and did then and there while drunk, attempt to supervise the arrangements of the sick in the said Hospital."[4]

Sanitary conditions at the post hospital were particularly offensive. Gross mismanagement of the sewage system had a domino effect. Defective drainpipes oozed sewage that surfaced near the hospital kitchen. Not only was food preparation tainted, but the waste "fill[ed] the air with offensive effluvia." Patients were moved to avoid the noxious influence. One ward was closed, which severely taxed the hospital's resources. The remaining hospital ward became severely overcrowded, adding to the collective misery. There were other hospital-related complaints. Medical officers decried the lack of a "dead house," and important autopsies were not performed for lack of space.[5]

News of the dismal situation at Alton finally leaked out, with blame for the deplorable state of affairs being placed squarely on the commander's shoulders. Colonel Weer was brought before a court-martial to answer for his mismanagement. The prosecutor filed five criminal charges containing a total of twenty-two specifications alleging misconduct. Colonel Weer defiantly pled not guilty to drunkenness, neglect of duty, conduct unbecoming an officer, disobeying a lawful command, and conduct to the prejudice of good order and military discipline.

When the trial opened, witnesses for the prosecution paraded forth, telling a tale of gross mismanagement, belligerent behavior, and excessive drinking. Colonel Weer countered each and every complaint. Backed into a corner, the colonel waged a feisty battle; his reputation was on the line.

The trial moved quickly. Even with the quick pace, Weer had not forgotten the hapless Major Stephens. The post commander's paranoia had clearly settled on Stephens. Believing that a coup was imminent, and that the major was the ringleader, Colonel Weer had taken preemptive action. He ordered the supposed traitor arrested. It was a desperate move hatched in an irrational moment, but, Stephens ultimately got his day in court at Colonel Weer's court-martial. His testimony was condemning.

When the evidence phase of the trial was concluded both sides anxiously awaited the verdict. The post commander had gallantly defended his integrity. The court-martial members listened, deliberated, and rendered a swift and decisive verdict. Colonel Weer was found guilty of many, but not all, of the twenty-two specifications. The former post commander enjoyed only a fleeting moment of vindication. Following the verdict, he was promptly cashiered from the service.

Military law proscribed drunkenness in the articles of war. Article 45 succinctly stated, "Any commissioned officer who shall be found drunk on his guard, party, or other duty, shall be cashiered. Any non-commissioned officer or soldier so offending shall suffer such corporeal punishment as shall be inflicted by the sentence of a court-martial."[6] As simple and straightforward as Article 45 was, innovative arguments defending misconduct were continually developed. This was probably a healthy development in the evolution of military law. The sheer number of alcohol-related offenses and the dire consequences of conviction were clearly an impetus to avoid that painful outcome. Novel legal defense strategies were used; some succeeded, while others failed. Through the exercise, a consensus defining Article 45 gradually developed strengthening the fair administration of military justice.

One legal defense in particular challenged the crime of being drunk while on "other duty." The vague definition of what constituted "other duty" fell to military courts to decipher, and there were different interpretations. The conservative opinion took a hard line: Military officers were always on duty. Proponents of this view insisted that operational readiness required full time allegiance. Such fidelity created an intriguing quandary. Could an officer, for example, be charged with misconduct under Article 45 if he became intoxicated at a social gathering? Even more worrisome was a potential prosecution flowing from an after-duty-hours intoxication in the privacy of military housing. The answers came from real cases.

A routine part of every officer's life was the duty roster, on which various jobs were rotated among a group of officers. Most were unpleasant impositions of one sort or another. "Officer of the day" was among that group of shared, disagreeable duties. This was not a particularly difficult job; most officers shouldered the responsibility easily. There was generally minimal social inconvenience. From observations before, during, and after the Civil War, Lt. Col. Stephen Vincent Benét authored, in 1868, *A Treatise on Military Law and the*

Practice of Courts-Martial, in which he provided both legal guidance and illustrative examples of complex legal issues. Benét tackled the military concept of drunkenness on duty by describing the case of "Captain S." As Benét's example would show, officers could attend a social gathering and still make themselves available for any military contingency. Captain S. tried to straddle duty and pleasure in that manner.[7] Unfortunately, Captain S. lost sight of the balance between the requirements of military duty and the pleasure of social discourse. According to Benét, Captain S. attended a party the same night he was assigned duty as officer of the day. It was apparently an opportunity the captain didn't want to miss. The captain attended the grand gala and enjoyed himself immensely, maybe too much. As the night wore on, the captain continued to drink heavily, and the alcohol took its toll as he grew giddy and silly. His rowdy behavior was like a magnet drawing embarrassed gazes in his direction. The steely disapproving eye of his commander signaled the end of the captain's riotous evening. He was finally hustled out, leaving a thankful group behind. The captain paid dearly for his debauch; he was arrested and charged with drunken misconduct under Article 45.

The court-martial members spent some time struggling over a definition of "official duty." Under normal circumstances, it seemed to stretch the limits of Article 45 to include an evening get-together. Unfortunately for the captain his assignment as officer of the day precluded much leeway. He was subsequently found guilty.

Benét provided another example of drunkenness on duty when he presented the case of "Lieutenant M." The story of Lieutenant M. expressed the worst nightmare many officers no doubt feared. Throughout the official workday officers were expected to abstain from alcohol or at least drink in moderation. Such sanctions did not seem to extend to off-duty hours, which was a commonsense rationalization that ignored the lengthy period of intoxication and withdrawal characteristic of alcohol consumption.

Lieutenant Colonel Benét recounted the story of Lieutenant M. to highlight the difficulty in rigidly applying the language of Article 45. Benét described an off-duty, late-night progressive state of intoxication that unfolded in the quarters of Lieutenant M. In this drowsy, confused condition the lieutenant acknowledged the vigorous knocking at his door. The lieutenant stumbled as he strode unsteadily across the room. As he tentatively opened the door, his blurred vision barely made out the indistinct image of a sergeant. The sergeant, speaking slowly because he recognized the lieutenant's condition, passed on an urgent order that required the lieutenant's immediate attention and response. Unfortunately, the lieutenant was unable to comply because of his drunken condition, which made the unit commander furious.

The lieutenant's court-martial for drunkenness focused on the familiar but vexing issue: Was it a military officer's obligation to be perpetually prepared for duty?[8] The trial-court was sympathetic, with court members accepting a boundary distinguishing the workday from private off-duty time. Barring obvious military obligations that would take precedence, this court-martial would not convict Lieutenant M. The lieutenant's drunkenness was judged to have occurred outside duty hours, and he was accordingly acquitted.

Legions of soldiers were prosecuted under Article 45. Disparate findings, based on similar circumstances, lent an air of capriciousness to the courts-martial process. The War Department vainly sought judicial explanations that would form the basis for unanimity. Exasperated, they finally issued clarifying directives. One government order issued in 1856, a scant four years before the Civil War, broadened the scope of what constituted military duty. Henceforth, any officer assigned a task where "he gets drunk after he has commenced it, and is thus rendered unable to continue it; or when having received an urgent and peremptory order . . . he is unable to execute it" will in all these cases be considered drunk on duty.[9]

The concept of continuous duty was not new. Certain positions, such as post commander and surgeon, obviously demanded this degree of readiness. Troops engaged in combat, or imminently expecting such, also bore the burden of constant vigil. An accused officer might decide it was hopeless to argue innocence based on the fact that he was off duty when he was drunk. There were other options.

The officer could directly challenge the claim by asserting he simply was not drunk. It was common knowledge that alcohol had different effects on people. Some "who held their liquor well" could drink copious, periodic, quantities without obvious impairment. Others maintained a more or less permanent state of alcohol indulgence, again, with minimal detriment.

Given the onerous criminal penalties for drunkenness, and the frequency of the offense, a pragmatic consensus gradually took hold. Clearly liquor flowed freely and soldiers imbibed to varying degrees. Intoxication was all too common, so as a consequence, legal drunkenness was considered something extraordinary, defined by nothing less than total stupefaction. This description of drunkenness was popular among the troops but drew criticism from military commanders. As commander of the Army of the Potomac, Maj. Gen. George B. McClellan commented, "Nothing can be more erroneous than to suppose that as long as an officer is not drunk to insensibility—a condition, moreover, in which he is far less apt to do mischief than when he is simply drunk enough to be indiscreet—he is not drunk at all. The fullest possession of his faculties, by every officer, is necessary to fit him to discharge his duties properly."[10]

Government orders were published over and over again endorsing McClellan's view. Courts-martial members were stubbornly unfazed. The resistance was formidable, even extending to the postwar years. In one case an officer was acquitted after jury members found "the accused was always more or less under the influence of alcohol, he never quite reached the gutter."[11] Another court-martial assessed drunkenness differently. Court-martial members who considered "a man must be in such a condition that he cannot ride" favorably disposed of this defendant's fate.[12] In this interpretation, short of falling out of the saddle, an officer was not drunk.

An enlisted soldier was not so lucky. Sgt. Thomas H. Blincoe, Company I, 2nd Cavalry, was assigned to the Department of the Pacific. In many units the use of whiskey was not only tolerated but also encouraged. Each man was, however, expected to drink responsibly. Sergeant Blincoe generally abided by this rule but unfortunately he drank a bit too much one day. Riding his horse through the dusty streets of Visalia, California, Blincoe suffered the embarrassment of falling off his mount. Embarrassment changed to shame when the sergeant's drunkenness became evident. This episode earned him a court-martial. The prosecution accused Sergeant Blincoe of "making himself a public spectacle to the disgrace of himself and company . . . [after getting] so drunk as to render himself unfit for duty."[13] The military jury spent very little time anguishing over Blincoe's case. He was found guilty and forced to begin his career anew as a private.

Alcohol was commonly prescribed as a medication. A cunning legal argument sought to explain drunkenness as a side effect from medicinal use. If the soldier could supplement his claim by appearing debilitated, so much the better. Testimony from a doctor was important if a defendant chose to use this defense, as the prosecution would surely contest the claim lacking such professional corroboration.[14]

Pvt. John Alexander had pulled guard duty for the second time in a week. Adding insult to injury, he shouldered the burden on Christmas Day. Army life had probably never been as exciting as he had expected. Drudgery, drills, and guard duty filled the days. Perhaps the combination of anger and disillusionment led him to the bottle for solace. When the appointed day for guard duty rolled around, Private Alexander toasted the holiday many times. His inebriation was obvious and the command response predictable. A court-martial was hastily convened. Private Alexander was accused of being "so under the influence of liquor as to be unable to perform the duty of a soldier."[15] He stood impassively as the sentence was read. "The Court after mature deliberation and the evidence adduced, find the accused, Private John Alexander, of Company 'D' Ninth U.S. Infantry . . . 'Guilty' of the charge; and does therefore sentence Private John Alexander . . . [t]o be confined at hard labor . . . for three months, wearing a twenty-four pound shot attached to his leg by a chain."

Punishments for drunkenness varied, ranging from extra duty to lengthy confinement or a dishonorable discharge. Every now and then first-time offenders, officers, or favorites were offered a special deal.

A soldier was bound by a code of honorable conduct, violation of which might forever damage his reputation, causing him to suffer public humiliation and to be shunned. This powerful influence was used to extract a promise of future good behavior from the soldier. When a formal written pledge was offered in lieu of punishment, there were legal ramifications.[16] Formal pledges were extended and accepted to avoid courts-martial, in some situations, averting the expense of trial and minimizing public embarrassment. Officers might offer the pledge "to avoid alcohol" to escape threatened punishment. A fairly well-documented postwar example illustrates the practice.

During the war complex, conflicting behaviors sometimes mixed with the freely available spirits, culminating in particularly vile military misconduct. The role alcohol played was variously debated in four courts-martial that nonetheless, each resulted in a death sentence.

Private James Weaver, alias N. E. Baker, suffered the ultimate penalty. Private Baker ran afoul of military authorities shortly after enlistment as a substitute in the First Regiment of the Maryland Volunteer Infantry.

The prosecution contended that Baker, along with two partners, bribed his way to freedom. New recruits were closely guarded after induction. That was a prudent measure since the reality of military life made it easier for many soldiers to disappear, but unofficial absences still rose to epidemic proportions. To combat this trend, newly enlisted soldiers were housed together in a common barracks, under the watchful eye of a guard. From this confined setting they would wait for assignment to their new units.

Private Baker and his two comrades desperately wanted out of the military. After weighing several options they settled on one possible ploy; perhaps they could bribe a guard. Their bold gamble paid off. Turning the guard's head was expensive, costing all of 140 dollars, yet the plan was still incomplete. The military uniform was an anchor bound to drag them down. A successful escape demanded civilian clothes, and somehow they acquired them. Without the civilian clothes, Private Baker could never have gotten a travel pass from the provost marshal. Despite his planning, Baker's absence was almost immediately detected, guaranteeing that his brief travel would turn out to be very costly. His itinerary extended from Ft. Monroe, Virginia, to Baltimore, Maryland. Three days into his adventure, he was abruptly seized aboard a U.S. mail boat.

Private Baker's court-martial was short and simple. The accused presented neither witnesses nor evidence, although a parade of prosecution witnesses testified. Their evidence was condemning. The defense rallied ineffectually, and a confrontation with a prosecution witness backfired. Whatever Private Baker's motives were, the consequence was the further admission of damning testimony. The witness Private Baker challenged had been duped into buying civilian clothes for the trio.

"He [Baker] told me there would be no difficulty about me buying the pants, I would be all right, that they were citizens—they handed their pants in a tent back of the jewelry store—they had on all citizens clothes except the pants at that time. They left their soldiers pants there, and I asked them what I should do with them. They told me I might have them. The pair of pants I have on belongs to this man, the prisoner. The prisoner here was the principal spokesman. . . ." The sole question put forth by the beleaguered lawbreaker was, "Did the prisoner give you . . . money?" "No sir . . ." was the unequivocal response.

Minimal repartee typified Baker's defense. He gained no ground during the trial. The last chance to turn a tide about to sweep him away depended on his final statement. The accused was given the privilege of addressing the jury just before they retired to consider the evidence. For many soldiers this personal plea amounted to their entire defense.

Private Baker faced the jury. "I am a native of Westmoreland, in the State of Virginia. I left there, that is Westmoreland, and came over to the federal lines and was sent to Washington, and there I took the oath of allegiance. I came over into these lines so as not to be conscripted into the Rebel services. After I took the oath, I went to Baltimore where I got work as a brakes man on the Baltimore and

Ohio Railroad. . . . I fell in company with a young man who said he was from the south. When I was in his company I thought myself perfectly safe, we got to drinking together, when I became in a state of intoxication—after I was with him for several hours, he induced me to enlist as a substitute. I was so intoxicated that I did not know what I was doing at that time . . . how I came into the service I was not aware. . . . I made inquiries about how I came there, no body could tell me, only that I came in there with a squad of other recruits. . . ." Baker ended his plea with a fervent prayer, "look into my case and do all you can for me and as I have no more defense to make I leave my care to the mercy of the court."

Private Baker's story rang with a tone of believability. Certain elements were plausible. Perhaps it was true that during a period of deep intoxication he made a poor choice and his Southern companion then took advantage of the situation. The natural skepticism of the court-martial members fed their doubt. Their first impulse was probably to dismiss Baker's story as a cleverly concocted tale to conceal his wrongdoing. Particularly damaging was the testimony about the plot to buy civilian clothes, behavior that was consistent with determined efforts to avoid detection and plan an escape. There were no defense witnesses, and when combined with a desultory cross-examination, the scales of justice tipped toward the prosecution. The verdict seemed inevitable. "After maturely deliberating upon the evidence adduced . . . ," Private Baker heard the verdict: He would face a squad armed with muskets and be shot. In less than three months, Private Baker had enlisted and deserted and was convicted and executed.[17]

Any good defense attorney abhors steamroller justice. A well-organized defense required witnesses, expert testimony, legal research, and if necessary, a thoughtful appeal. Private Baker, guilty or not, had none of these. Baker's case was typical of the time, exposing inadequacies in the administration of military justice that fueled a perception of inequity.

The case of Pvt. Henry Holt, Company F, 2nd New Hampshire Volunteers, was more complex. The charge was desertion, although Private Holt would introduce some novel arguments against that charge. Even so, alcohol played the central role in his defense. Holt had joined the Union effort with the best of intentions. It was a proud November day for him, when he was mustered into service. The following few months revealed a soldier with promise, not distinguished in performance, but possessing a good character. Private Holt was young, and his impressionable spirit that absorbed patriotic virtues was also vulnerable to vices. Holt's moral decline began shortly after he left home. Temptations lurked everywhere, but the easiest to indulge came corked in a bottle. The alcohol seemed to have a corrosive effect on Private Holt's personality. He grew increasingly weary of Army discipline and the monotonous routine. His fellow soldiers noticed a slow deterioration in his work. Eventually, Holt's only pursuit was drinking, and four months after induction, Private Holt missed roll call while stationed in Yorktown, Virginia. Hardly anyone was surprised.

Private Holt enjoyed forty-eight hours of freedom, until an alert and suspicious mail boat captain terminated his absence. Holt was spotted, along with two others, lazily floating down the York River in a small open boat, apparently appropriated more for convenience than concealment. That was a fatal mistake. Desertion ran rampant in the Union Army, and public-minded citizens considered it a matter of civic responsibility to staunch the flow. The mail boat captain spied the men drifting down river from an Army camp, and when he hailed the young sailors, there was no response. The silence seemed to deepen the captain's suspicions that these men were deserters. A warning shot fired from the mail boat brought the intrepid soldiers about, and they were all arrested. Private Holt and his companions had traveled about twenty miles from their unit. The trip back was quicker and far less pleasant.

Private Holt was accused of desertion, and his trial was marked by brevity. He pled guilty and offered little in the way of a conventional defense; however, his statement to the court provided some explanation of his behavior. Holt, unconvincingly and apparently without passion, admitted, "drinking very freely." Stimulated through immoderation, Private Holt "took a small boat and went down one of the creeks into the Bay." He vigorously denied a key criminal element of desertion: the intent to permanently leave his unit. In fact, Holt cleverly stressed just the opposite. His excursion had been a temporary lark to show his good faith. Private Holt proposed that he "pay all expenses . . . be restored to his Company, and . . . be a good soldier in the future."

The court-martial members were in no frame of mind to negotiate. They did not believe Holt's cock-and-bull story. Jury deliberations were perfunctory—there was after all very little evidence to consider. The court-martial members returned after a brief recess, finding Private Holt guilty of desertion and sentenced to "be shot to death with musketry, in the presence of his regiment."

Holt's day of doom was delayed for several weeks, his fate in the hands of President Lincoln. The judge advocate general's office took the offensive role and, in a letter to the President, set forth his objections to clemency: "While intoxication, or other causes that prevent the full use of the mental faculties, may properly be inquired into and considered for the purpose of ascertaining the intervention of a soldier, in absenting himself in this manner, it is sufficient to say that in this case, there is no evidence whatever as to the condition of the prisoner in these respects at the time he is charged to have committed this offense." President Lincoln read the judge advocate's report carefully. The reasoning was sound. Aside from alcohol, there were no other mitigating factors. The sentence was approved, and Pvt. Henry Holt was executed.[18]

The criminal case involving Larkin W. Ray, a private in Company C of the 7th Kentucky Volunteer Infantry, was a complex tale. Alcohol played a central role in the drama as well as a lack of counsel for the accused.

The Sun Billiard Saloon was a favorite destination of Union soldiers stationed at Baton Rouge, Louisiana. Mr. P. Billard, the keeper of the saloon, tried not to mix politics with his liquor. Success kept his saloon open and busy. Scattered about the room were numerous well-worn tables and chairs. Several billiard tables in similar condition promised a distracting recreation for the patrons. The noise level flowed in a predictable manner. As the day wore on, a crescendo steadily built with each new arrival until the placed loudly buzzed. At this point, Mr. Billard would open the door to his saloon, having learned that this cacophony attracted passersby.

Calamity struck Baton Rouge early in the evening on the second of December 1864. The sun had just set, and soldiers freed from duty were gravitating toward the saloons. Saloons like the Sun Billiard were more than just drinking establishments—they were social hubs. Officers mingled with each other, as did enlisted soldiers, yet, despite the relaxed environment, military rules of etiquette generally frowned on familiarities being exchanged between officers and enlisted soldiers.

Dr. W. K. Sadler was assigned to the 19th Kentucky Volunteer Infantry and held the position of Surgeon in Chief of the Military District of Baton Rouge and Port Hudson. After an arduous day attending medical responsibilities, Dr. Sadler retired to the Sun Billiard Room. The saloonkeeper recognized the genial surgeon, and, after exchanging pleasantries, Dr. Sadler took his drink and absently began watching a billiard game in progress. His reverie was rudely disturbed.

Pvt. Larkin W. Ray enjoyed simple pleasures. Beer and whiskey were the cheapest, and best, recreational pursuits. Joined by a friend, Pvt. Lewis Roarch, Company D, 7th Kentucky Volunteer Infantry, the two soldiers indulged freely that night. Neither got stumbling drunk, but both were emboldened, irritable, and tactless. The pair sampled several saloons and, in the process, they became increasingly boisterous. In this condition, the two soldiers entered the Sun Billiard Room.

Private Ray and his friend stormed into the small saloon. The saloonkeeper read their behavior and saw trouble. They were bent on making mischief. Moving from table to table, Ray and his friend made their obnoxious, intrusive presence felt. At one point Ray gathered up the billiard balls from an active game and tossed them about. The howl of protest motivated Military Surgeon Sadler to intervene. Identifying himself as a military officer, Sadler sternly ordered the two frolicsome soldiers into a brief composure. Ray's friend, smarting from the rebuke, angrily took a seat in the corner.

A small party of officers led by Capt. E. Trulon of the 2nd Louisiana Infantry entered the Sun Billiard Room a few moments later, unaware of the earlier fracas. The party's casual, lighthearted manner offered the perfect foil for the recently chastised privates. Jousting began when Ray's friend, with thinly veiled contempt, approached the officers and truculently proclaimed "he did not care . . . for any citizen, officer, or soldier." This unprovoked comment delivered with angry affect stunned the officers into momentary silence. One of the officers finally asked what regiment Private Ray's friend belonged to. Before the question was answered, another officer noted the private's "tight" condition and counseled his friends to ignore the intoxicated soldier.

Captain Trulon turned his attention to Ray, cautioning "that if he was a soldier he probably knew his duty and that was not to interfere with officers." Private Ray was further instructed to gather up his friend and return to quarters. The chastened soldier grudgingly acknowledged his general respect for military officers but unfortunately, a drunken loyalty to his friend forced a belligerent comeback. A heated exchange followed. Tiring of the process, Trulon preempted further arguments by asserting, "if you remain here and continue quarreling, you will get into trouble."

While Private Ray and Captain Trulon were arguing, Ray's friend was spoiling for a fight. Approaching a young lieutenant, Private Ray's friend issued a loud insult, "I don't think you are an officer." Following a short, sharp exchange, the young lieutenant exploded and, uttering an oath, he grabbed Private Ray's friend and threw him out of the billiard room. During the scuffle, Private Ray's friend threw a brick at the lieutenant. The missile fell harmlessly to the floor. Ray's friend was forcefully evicted, and Ray continued his misguided support of his friend by complaining to the lieutenant "that, that man was a friend of his and that he would not see him abused."

The young lieutenant, still excited from the recent provocation, had sufficient energy left for Ray. Proclaiming his authority as an officer, the lieutenant screamed that "he was an officer and would take no such talk from a Private soldier." Private Ray was similarly ejected from the Sun Billiard Room. One of the privates ominously promised revenge.

This incident upset Captain Trulon and his fellow officers and they left the saloon. The innkeeper barred the door after them, fearing a return of the truculent soldiers. When Billard locked his door the only patrons remaining behind were the military surgeon and a Mr. Edwards.

Billard's worst fears were realized when about fifteen minutes later a thunderous pounding on the door shook the saloon. The barkeeper's first impulse was to ignore the noise. A brief discussion passed between Billard and the congenial surgeon. The surgeon persuaded Billard to open the door.

Surgeon Sadler put on his uniform coat, as Private Ray and his friend quickly reentered the saloon. They were armed with a musket, which they menacingly pointed at the surgeon. There seemed to be little fear in Sadler as he strode self-assuredly forward. Within a few paces of Ray the surgeon stopped and asked the pair what their intentions were. Ray tried to dismiss Sadler by ordering him out of the saloon, but the surgeon resisted. A shot rang out, and Sadler "folded his arms around his body" and slumped toward the ground, after which both soldiers fled. The barkeeper did his best to comfort Sadler in his remaining moments of his life.

Private Ray mustered virtually no defense at his subsequent court-martial, although it probably wouldn't have mattered much anyway. The murder of an officer and physician evoked little sympathy. After a short deliberation, the jury sentenced Pvt. Larkin W. Ray "to be hanged by the neck, until he is dead . . . in the presence of as many Troops at that post as the exigencies of the service will permit."[19]

First Sgt. Darius Philbrooks, Company K, 1st Regiment, Colored Volunteers, was charged as follows: "[O]n the 13th day of March 1862, [drew] a pistol on Lieutenant Isaac Gray, First Colorado Volunteers, and shot said Lieutenant Gray." Philbrooks's court-martial was significant in one respect—according to the official list of U.S. Soldiers Executed during the Civil War, Philbrooks was one of a few men holding a higher rank to be sentenced to death. Despite his rank, Philbrooks gained no advantage during his court-martial; he was still left to his own resources in defending himself.

Mr. Emanuel Spiegelberg operated a sutler's store near Ft. Union, New Mexico, in 1862. Closely attached to this mercantile establishment was a small house, and the business and lodging were suitable for both Mr. Spiegelberg and a porter he employed. The sutler's store supplied the territory with essential goods and served as a social hub. Soldiers, trappers, and other local civilians depended on the sutler's store for recreation too. Occasionally, the owner would reward his customers by hosting a "formal" gathering, which attracted the attention of patrons throughout the local area. These were good-natured affairs that strengthened community bonds. Of course, the goodwill translated into more business for the sutler.

The uneasy relationship between the military and sutlers who sold alcohol was expressed by Article 29. Sutlers were strictly prohibited from selling liquor after 9:00 P.M., before reveille, or during the Sunday sermon.

First Sergeant Philbrooks heard about one of the sutler's community gatherings by word of mouth. The event promised to be a pleasing diversion from the monotony of camp routine. Having a fondness for intoxicants, the first sergeant was particularly attracted by the promise of free-flowing liquor.

Philbrooks had ten years of military service—good years, by most accounts. His record of service was sufficient to justify a series of promotions, but his decade of service was not trouble free. Philbrooks was the first to admit that his prior difficulties were entirely suffered "through indulgence with liquor." A tolerant military command discounted these indiscretions as an understandable consequence of a hard life. Perhaps this collusion by command insulated the sergeant.

Sergeant Philbrooks was a good soldier, except when he was drunk. His regiment clearly minimized the sergeant's periodic belligerence, perhaps considering alcohol the culprit and not the man. The relationship between this senior noncommissioned officer and his commanders surely fostered an implicit agreement. A subtle contract allowed the first sergeant a certain free reign. In exchange for loyal duty, a few alcohol-related gaffes were overlooked. Years of collusion had reinforced the pact. The arrangement might have survived except for one fatal miscalculation: By always escaping serious punishment Philbrooks probably never saw the need to cut down on his drinking, and, with no constraints forcing moderation, a reckless course of escalation seemed inevitable.

First Sergeant Philbrooks arrived at the sutler's house early in the evening, yet despite his early arrival, the house was crowded. The first sergeant liberally helped himself to the liquor. As the intoxicating spirits slowly dissolved his better judgment, Philbrooks grew increasingly rambunctious. Mr. Spiegelberg's porter was embarrassed by the first sergeant's indecorous behavior and complained to his employer. Spiegelberg listened with concern to his porter, but remained insufficiently motivated to intervene, perhaps figuring that his unruly guest would settle down. Spiegelberg briefly left the noisy crowd and puttered about his store, making minor preparations for the next business day. An exasperated interruption by his porter again forced to his attention the intemperate behavior of the first sergeant. The porter had spotted Philbrooks with a "quart tin cup about half filled with liquor." The porter's message was clear: This soldier was drunk enough. The storeowner could not ignore further indulgence, in light of Philbrooks's already obnoxious state.

Mr. Spiegelberg was determined; striding forcefully over to First Sergeant Philbrooks, the sutler pointed at the cup of liquor and expressed his sternest disapproval. Philbrooks summoned forth what indignation his drunken mind allowed. The liquor was "not all for me," the surprised soldier exclaimed, he planned "to treat a few friends." The sutler was on the verge of an angry response, when a nearby officer intervened.

The verbatim transcript of Philbrooks's trial introduced the sworn testimony of a Lt. Isaac Gray next. Gray had joined the happy crowd at the sutler's home earlier in the evening. Socializing with others was always an enjoyable pastime for him. As an officer, Lieutenant Gray naturally expected certain rules of propriety to govern any social affair. First Sergeant Philbrooks had captured Lieutenant Gray's attention, not only because of his rank, but also because of his boisterous manner. Although the two knew each other, Gray clearly concluded that this soldier was an embarrassment.

Lieutenant Gray felt obligated to admonish the reckless soldier, and his opportunity came, when the sutler unsuccessfully confronted Sergeant Philbrooks. Seizing the initiative, Gray asserted his authority and invited the drunken soldier to leave, but the sutler was the only person to leave.

Emboldened by the liquor, First Sergeant Philbrooks argued with his superior instead of obeying him. For a few minutes the two sparred verbally. Recognizing the futility of further words, Gray sought to forcibly evict Philbrooks. The first sergeant swore violently and resisted physically. Sensing the need for reinforcements, the officer threatened to call military guards for assistance, and the warning had a momentary calming effect on Philbrooks. Briefly in control of the situation, Lieutenant Gray escorted the drunken soldier out the door.

Philbrooks was humiliated. His passions ignited by the fiery liquor, Philbrooks sought revenge not more than ten yards from the site of his public disgrace. Secretly withdrawing his holstered pistol, the first sergeant took deliberate aim and shot Lieutenant Gray. More stunned than injured, Gray unsheathed his sword and viciously struck at Philbrooks. Although Gray managed to injure Philbrooks, it was an unequal match. The first sergeant fired again, knocking Lieutenant Gray to the ground.

Despite his drunken state, the first sergeant must have recognized the gravity of his offense, causing him to flee the area, but his escape was observed and pistols were drawn. Several shots were fired in a vain attempt to stop him; the bullets went wide of their mark, but the poor aim did not benefit the first sergeant. Intoxication, the sword wound, and fear combined to trip up the fleeing felon. Philbrooks was lying prostrate on the ground when a Captain Logan approached him.

The captain had witnessed the fracas and was among those who fired at Philbrooks. A cursory examination proved that Philbrooks was not seriously injured, and he was promptly arrested. His court-martial was convened shortly thereafter.

The prosecutor had a strong case. The sutler would provide graphic testimony describing the accused's belligerent behavior. He was an eyewitness to all events except the shooting. Another witness for the prosecution was Surgeon H. I. Peck of the 4th New Mexico Volunteers, who had provided medical care to Lieutenant Gray. The surgeon described the wound as "a pistol ball passed between both eyes, a little above—the Ball passed through the bones of the nose into which is called the posterior chamber of that organ." Remarkably, Dr. Peck predicted "that he will recover from the wound inflicted on him." The doctor's dramatic testimony was the perfect place to conclude the prosecution's case. Left lingering in the mind of the court-martial members was the picture of a wantonly crippled officer.

First Sergeant Philbrooks was a fighter. Ten years of military service had left its mark. He had been in scrapes before and had always managed his way out. The first sergeant was determined to wage a spirited defense. Believing that his alcohol-related misadventures had been overlooked before and could be yet again, it was little wonder that Philbrooks conducted his own defense, marshaled his own witnesses, and sought to evade consequences by blaming his friend—the bottle.

Sergeant Philbrooks called E. M. Quimby, Company K, 1st Colorado Volunteers, as his first witness. Unfazed by his new role as a defense attorney, the feisty first sergeant interrogated Quimby, "Was I sober or not at the time the occurrence happened between Lieutenant Gray and myself?" Quimby failed to answer the question directly, instead, providing a good character reference of the first sergeant based on their lengthy relationship. "I never knew him to be in a difficulty of this kind before." Quimby's effectiveness was watered down when a court member asked when was the last time the pair had been stationed together. Captain Quimby confessed that he had had no contact with the prisoner for the last seven years.

The second defense witness was 2nd Lt. R. S. Underhill. Echoing Quimby, the junior officer expressed profound faith and confidence in the accused. "He was a non commissioned officer of very high standards . . . and I have never known him to be in any difficulty before this time." This untainted testimony must have pleased the accused. Sergeant Philbrooks attacked the heart of the prosecution's case with this witness. The accused soldier hoped to wear down the standing of prosecution witnesses with his own eyewitness. It was a chancy strategy. This important eyewitness began his testimony by declaring that Philbrooks "was not sober" while at the sutler's home. This line of inquiry animated the jury members, and they seemed to pounce in unison. Stealing the initiative from the first sergeant, the jury members silenced the accused by co-opting his witness. They were not concerned with the prisoner's venture into an alcohol-related excuse. "Did you see the prisoner fire at Lieutenant Gray?" one of the jury members pointedly asked. The witness, after a moment's reflection, answered, "I saw him draw his pistol, but could not say he fired." Another court member wondered "when the prisoner drew his pistol did he make any remark in an angry manner?" Sergeant Philbrook's witness responded simply, "I did not hear him."

Philbrooks's last witness was 2nd Lt. J. H. Dawson, 1st Colorado Volunteers. The lieutenant was another character reference well suited to comment on the defendant's recent duty performance. "I always considered him one of the best Orderly Sergeants we had in the Regiment, and never knew of anything in his conduct, but what was gentlemanly and soldierly—the present difficulty to my knowledge is the first he has been in, since my acquaintance with him."

Philbrooks concluded his defense with a short, impassioned plea for clemency, beginning with the frank admission that he was incapable of overcoming the temptation of the bottle. The first sergeant added a touch of remorse to his confession, lamenting his victim's injury. "I am very sorry that I have got into a difficulty with Lieutenant Gray, as I always looked upon him as one of my best friends. I was drunk when the occurrence took place, and I scarcely recollect anything that occurred at the time."

Sergeant Philbrooks conducted a reasonable defense. He challenged elements of the prosecution's case, buttressed his position with several good character references, acknowledged his weakness with liquor, and apologized. Some might have thought the fact that Gray was expected to survive might have been a plus in favor of the defendant. The jury considered his fate for only a short time. The fact that jury members had telegraphed an ominous disdain for drunkenness when they derailed the testimony of one of Philbrooks' witnesses was a clue to the outcome.

The court-martial convicted Sergeant Philbrooks and by a two-thirds vote sentenced him to "be shot to death at such time and manner as the Commanding Officer of the Department . . . may direct." For the first time, Philbrooks's justifications failed. The bill for ten years' worth of credit for alcohol-related misconduct came due, and was paid in full.

Sergeant Philbrooks was fundamentally a good soldier who, through poor judgment, had carelessly inflicted injury. He clearly lacked an incorrigibly malevolent life history. Nonetheless, Sergeant Philbrooks was harshly judged. Courts-martial members were swayed perhaps by several factors, one of which, of course, was the fact that twice Philbrooks resorted to the use of firearms and grievously wounded an officer. Philbrooks was a senior member of the military and was surely held to a higher standard of behavior than enlisted men, given his years of service.[20]

Alcohol was obviously a major problem during the Civil War. Commissary stores stocked whiskey, but even without that resource, nonmilitary sources were abundant. Ease of access and ambivalent rules regarding use contributed partly to abuse. The official statistics compiled from field medical reports surely underestimated alcoholism. These reports tabulated alcohol abuse under three banners: inebriation, delirium tremens, and chronic alcoholism.[21] Numbers were higher at the beginning of the war. Proximity to urban centers inflated the numbers, reflecting in part the easier access. Imperfect definitions of alcohol abuse and a tendency to ignore the diagnosis contributed to the unrealistic official numbers. The War Department reported an average of 4.6 cases of inebriation, delirium tremens, and chronic alcoholism per one thousand white troops annually. According to the official reports only an astonishing half percent of soldiers ever got drunk. Court-martial records, government orders, and soldier's diaries seemed to contest the official line. These sources were chock-full of entries documenting alcohol-related misconduct. The annual rate reported among colored troops was a minuscule 0.22 per thousand. Among white troops only one case out of 220 officially received medical attention.[22]

The Union Army numbered in excess of a million volunteers for the entire war effort. The vast majority was between eighteen and forty-five years old, with the average age around twenty-five.[23] More than three-quarters were native-born Americans. A large contingent of German-born troops supplemented the Union ranks, followed in numbers by the Irish. Both groups enjoyed strong drinks. From this vast assemblage of young men, about only one thousand medical reports of inebriation were submitted each year.

The official records stood in stark contrast to the recorded accounts of disciplinary problems. Alcohol-related problems predictably peaked when soldiers were paid. Even commissary whiskey, generally shunned by soldiers because of its presumed poor quality, was eagerly consumed. Typical consequences followed as rowdy troops filled guardhouses.

The official government numbers minimized the negative impact of alcohol, but reality prevented most commanders the luxury of turning a blind eye. The most ardent among that group waged a moral war; a relatively informal network developed between these officers, chaplains, and temperance advocates to promote abstinence. Various measures were enlisted, ranging in intensity from fiery, condemning sermons, to surprise inspections, denying civilian peddlers access to military posts, and declaring nearby cities off-limits to troops. The tension between advocates of this broad social reform movement who sought to outlaw inebriation inevitably collided with those who held more moderate views. Many hard-drinking military soldiers probably considered those efforts misguided, particularly when the harsh realities of war were softened by a swig of whiskey.

A high-level Army investigation uncovered a unique approach some officers employed in the war against drunkenness. The scheme was uncovered when complaints from troops surfaced in the District of West Florida. The appearance of scurvy among the soldiers was a frightening discovery that added concern to the complaints. Military investigators were amazed by what they discovered—a totally corrupt food sharing system. Officers were liberally spending money to procure fresh food and libations for themselves. However, the largess was not shared, proving once again that rank definitely had its privileges—to the detriment of the enlisted men. Nowhere was the imbalance more pronounced than with the whiskey. The District of West Florida was authorized a monthly allocation in September of 2,345 gallons of whiskey. Officers reserved for their personal use almost two gallons a month, whereas the troops enjoyed far less, not even a cup of spirits a month. An unintended consequence was a reduction in fisticuffs among the enlisted troops. The military investigators restored equity.[24]

Major General George B. McClellan complained early in the war "drunkenness is the cause of by far the greater part of the disorders which are examined by the courts-martial."[25] Drunkenness was such a common offense, in spite of the official records, that convening courts-martial in each instance was impractical. Commanders resorted to summary judgment, a practical option that spared the commander the trouble of assembling a trial. Evidence was gathered informally and the decision quickly reached. A common punishment for overindulgence was confinement in a guard tent.[26] A brief period of restricted liberty seemed fair.

Some troops still never learned; the lure of the bottle was too great. Couple that with a teetotaling commander, and novel penalties cropped up. Pvt. Patrick Bolen, toward the end of the conflict in 1864, was known throughout the camp for his intemperate manner. Ignoring, condoning, excusing, or ridiculing his besotted behavior were ineffective deterrents. Private Bolen was branded throughout the camp as a habitual drunk. He became such an embarrassment that no alternative remained but to take legal action. The court-martial members used the occasion to send two messages, one for Bolen and the other to his unit. Patrick Bolen was convicted of habitual drunkenness. The punishment imposed was "to have one side of his head shaved, and in the presence of the Battalion be drummed out of service, with a stoppage of all pay and allowances."[27] Bolen suffered the immediate shame, but it was hoped that future malefactors could avoid the same fate.

Military law operated under the premise that voluntarily intoxication exposed the drinker to a risk.[28] He could indulge as his whim dictated but would be held responsible for any indignities. A schism existed in assessing moral culpability, though. One group insisted that all alcohol-related crimes deserved extra punishment. The willful consumption of the mind-altering substance was, in itself, considered negligent. According to members of this persuasion, alcohol was an aggravating factor that justified greater punishment.

In general practice, intoxication was commonly presented as an excuse for misconduct.[29] The accused soldiers hoped to mitigate punishment, which increased the probability of a counterfeit claim. That nagging suspicion lurked in the background of many a courts-martial member's mind.

Capt. Richard Lee was weary. His dream of battle-won glory had conflicted harshly with the ugly realities of combat. People were killed and maimed with alarming frequency. Training, group cohesion, and inner strength helped to suppress this normal fear, and weak-kneed soldiers had to weigh the disgrace and the punishment of succumbing to fear. Captain Lee grappled daily with a moral dilemma: Fight and die, or run and live. Malingering was a creative solution that seemed to bridge the chasm between these two conflicting positions.

Captain Lee undoubtedly reasoned that any method he chose to induce self-harm must be transient, painless and with a nondetectable cause. He accomplished the first two criteria, but he should have spent more time perfecting his ruse. His effort to feign illness was clumsy. Captain Lee wanted a quick and easy way to get sick, and to minimize suffering, a short recovery. His goal, after all, was merely to avoid the pending deployment. A noxious combination of chewing tobacco, alcohol, "and other means" caused Lee to become violently ill, but the charade was uncovered. Perhaps a fellow officer hinted that Captain Lee was faking or the surgeon recognized the pungent smell of the alcohol-tobacco concoction and grew suspicious. In any event, Captain Lee was hauled into a military courtroom.

The prosecutor claimed that Captain Lee while "in command of the Regiment . . . chew[ed] tobacco, and used other means to make himself sick in a cowardly manner, that he might have an excuse for avoiding the coming engagement with the enemy."[30]

There were six specifications charging Captain Lee with cowardice before the enemy. Concerns, founded or otherwise, that bogus illness was rampant held sway with many officers. Overt evidence of an officer malingering confirmed that belief. This was an opportunity for court members to express repugnance, and, as a consequence, they dismissed Captain Lee from the Army.

An attorney preparing a legal defense of alcohol-related misconduct could turn to several authorities. Of particular value were medical theories purporting to explain personality and a propensity to develop certain human frailties such as alcoholism. At the time phrenology, the belief that mental faculties and character could be determined by "reading" the surface of the skull, was a dominant theory of human behavior.[31] Consultants in phrenology routinely advised enlightened mental hospital directors, prison wardens, and the general medical community; however, over time, some of phrenology's shine was lost. Scientific scrutiny steadily chipped away at phrenology's ideas. Despite the decline of phrenology in general, one of its tenets survived: the supposed correlation between physiognomy and criminal behavior.

Isaac Ray was a general medical practitioner in the small, rural village of Eastport, Maine, who was captivated by phrenology as it related to crime. His later clinical experience gravitated toward the treatment of mentally ill offenders. Years of work and personal study were distilled in an important book: *A Treatise on the Medical Juris-prudence of Insanity*, first published in 1838.[32]

Medical testimony was occasionally admitted as evidence in civil-ian trials, but rarely in courts-martial. A physician's contribution was generally limited to matters considered outside the experience of an average person. Opinions regarding the effects of alcohol, for example, were firmly within the bounds of lay knowledge. No expert testimony was needed. After all, drinking too much reflected a moral deficiency, not a medical problem. While not fully dismissing the weak character of an alcoholic, Isaac Ray believed that medical explanations also existed for drunkenness. The search for justice demanded that jury members hear this new line of thinking. Isaac Ray dramatized alco-hol-related criminal malfeasance with clinical vignettes.

Alexander Drew was a decent commander, and sailors appreci-ated his even-tempered, fair administration. For this, considerable lat-itude was given to his one weakness—"the excessive use of ardent spirits."[33] Even so, complaints mounted and Drew's stock of goodwill dissipated more rapidly than his supply of liquor. The captain recog-nized his plummeting favor among the crew, and, with an eye toward restoring his position, he resorted to a very public ploy. His private hoard of liquor was tossed overboard. This ship would sail dry.

The officers and crew were delighted with Alexander Drew's resolve. Better days lay ahead—or so the beleaguered crew hoped. A few days later, the captain complained of disturbed sleep and poor appetite. The crew took notice but attached no particular significance to the complaints. What followed riveted the ship's complement.

Drew unsteadily strolled the deck, muttering to himself, and his behavior alarmed the crew. They caught disturbing snatches of Drew's ramblings. The captain was convinced his life was threatened and that someone on board wanted to kill him. Standing in contrast to this suspiciousness were violent mood swings. At times the captain was ebullient, often singing in a loud, raucous voice, then, just as sud-denly, he would shift to a somber recitation of hymns.

Charles Clark served as Drew's second mate, and, as an officer, he had frequent opportunities to witness this erratic behavior. On one occasion, Clark was enjoying his morning repast when Drew belligerently ordered him up on deck. Just the night before, Drew had nearly jumped overboard, and quick action by the observant crew had saved him. Clark demurred, offering to go up on deck after he had finished his breakfast. His second mate's dismissive attitude apparently incensed the captain, and, somewhat impulsively, Drew pulled out a hidden knife and stabbed Clark. Remarkably, despite a mortal wound, Clark climbed to the upper deck, where, shortly thereafter, he died.

Drew followed the dying second mate, and standing imperiously before his stunned crew, ordered the ship ashore. The chief mate ignored the order, and retaining a presence of mind, instead had his commander confined. During the next few weeks, as the ship returned home, the captain suffered periods of maniacal behavior. During one of his more sedate moments, the officers had a chance to question their captain. Genuine perplexity and remorse was the best Drew could muster—he didn't remember anything.

Drew's trial for murder examined a novel supposition: Can a person plagued by habitual drunkenness, but temporarily abstinent, succumb to insanity? As the court noted, "[If] Drew was in a fit of intoxication, he would have been liable to be convicted of murder. As he was not then intoxicated, but merely insane from an abstinence from liquor, he cannot be pronounced guilty."[34]

Cases like that of Alexander Drew piqued Isaac Ray's interest and inspired him to study the influence of alcohol in a new light. Ray recognized that popular opinion cast a jaundiced eye on excusing alcohol-related misconduct. His goal was to introduce new medical knowledge to a jury. It began with a review of the levels of intoxication, which introduced a new idea. "The first effect of alcoholic liquors is to exalt the general sentiment of self-satisfaction and diffuse an unusual serenity over the mind. . . . Soon the torrent of his ideas becomes more rapid and violent, and he can scarcely repress them. This is the moment of his happiest sallies. . . . As yet the brain is in tolerable order . . . (although) thoughts succeed one another too rapidly to allow sufficient time to arrange them. . . . As the alcohol takes a firmer grip on mental facilities . . . his sensations lose their ordinary delicacy . . . he now feels an irresistible propensity to talk nonsense, but is perfectly conscious all the while that it is nonsense. . . . His imagination is filled by strange and queer images. . . . He is apt to imagine he has offended someone . . . or that he has been offended, and fixes upon someone as the object of his maledictions, perhaps his blows." According to Ray the deterioration deepens, and irrational thinking takes firm hold of the mental faculties. Soon drunkenness reaches its point of peak impairment.[35]

Repeatedly bathing the brain in alcohol has other consequences. The alcoholic begins to favor the company of the bottle at the expense of his friends, and he starts to avoid the community of his fellowman. A compulsive urge to drink relentlessly usurps willpower, and this destruction of willpower is coupled with a physiologic change. Ray was convinced that chronic alcohol ingestion altered normal brain function. He offered this medical model to counter traditional moral explanations of habitual drunkenness. Ray concluded, "The drunkenness being thus an accidental, involuntary consequence of a maniacal state of the mind, it cannot impart the character of criminality to any action to which it may give rise."[36]

The major contribution Isaac Ray added to the medical-legal discussion of alcoholism was to offer a medical, less moral, etiological explanation for the disorder. It would be many years following Ray's early observations before a basic fact about alcohol was widely accepted; that being the physiologic effects of alcohol, which persist long after consumption ceases. In fact, acute alcohol withdrawal precipitates a host of life-threatening and mind-altering consequences. Alexander Drew's behavior typified the state of alcohol withdrawal, a condition Isaac Ray noted, but didn't fully understand.

For a defense attorney this enlightened concept of habitual drunkenness was useful. Perhaps an impressive physician could sway a jury. An attorney of the Civil War era probably had little confidence that erudite medical testimony would influence a court-martial, since alcohol abuse was far too common a problem. Its use was connected with innumerable instances of malingering and malfeasance. Alcohol was just too convenient an excuse.

During the early days of the war effort, company officers were elected by their troops, and the officers in turn selected their superiors. In theory, this egalitarian approach promised a democratic bliss; however, in practice, officers were selected on popularity, not military competence. The system promoted patronage and in some respects held command hostage to the whims of the voters. Leaders in Washington recognized the danger, eventually transferring authority to commission officers to the state governors. Embedded in the transfer of power was statutory language creating a review panel. The new law formed "a military board or commission of not less than three nor more than five officers, whose duty it shall be to examine the capacity, qualifications, propriety of conduct, and efficiency of any commissioned officer." The board had the power to strip an officer's commission. Many of these military examination boards were mired in controversy.[37]

Although the military examination board was created exclusively to eliminate unwarranted influence, its success in that endeavor was questionable. Supporters argued that military examination boards raised overall standards, but there was no proof to support that contention. Lacking real proof of effectiveness, supporters nonetheless claimed that incompetent candidates weeded themselves out. They were afraid of being humiliated by the board and consequently avoided submitting an application. The military probably benefited by this self-screening process.

Routine board examination procedure varied. Flexibility, lack of structure, and an absence of uniform guidance contributed to an appearance of inconsistency. Experience eventually created better functioning boards. Examinations tested prospective officers on tactics, regulations, and moral fitness. "Gross immorality, habitual drunkenness, keeping low company, shirking duty, undue familiarity with subordinates, or incapacity to govern men will be considered as disqualifications."[38] Those not making the grade the first time were often allowed a second chance.

The board determined moral fitness by reading testamentary letters. Occasionally, a board would query candidates directly, although such scrutiny was the exception. Particularly egregious were instances when moral fitness was doubted but the board turned a blind eye. The effectiveness of military examination boards suffered from the same ills it sought to correct: political intrusion, prejudice, and a reluctance to confront identified shortcomings.

Particularly disheartening were instances of malfeasance among medical doctors. Even without misconduct, military physicians were frequently objects of derision. Primitive medical knowledge, combined with a general ignorance of military procedures, dealt a double blow to their image. Early in the war, a respected government agency, after examining two hundred regimental surgeons, concluded that 20 percent were incompetent, and another 20 percent received only a grudging nod of approval.[39] A sizable number of those failing to pass muster did so because of their intemperate habits.

Alcohol was a common medicinal agent. In the therapeutic setting, alcohol offered attractive benefits that included anesthesia and a mind-altering euphoria. The former promised to blunt the pain of surgical operations, while the latter provided relief, not necessarily cure, for a host of maladies. Intemperate doctors were well situated to exploit their medical stocks. This occupational hazard further blighted the reputation of medical care.

One surgeon, making a public spectacle of his drunkenness, "went staggering through the camp . . . with one man on each side of him." He compounded his personal disgrace through medical negligence. The doctor left his post and returned home, totally ignoring the suffering of the patients he abandoned. They were left without "a particle of medicine, food, delicacies." Another medical officer combined habitual drunkenness with cowardice. This surgeon left his sick and wounded soldiers to fend for themselves, while he sought a safer refuge from combat. He was later court-martialed and dismissed from the military.[40]

Several reports surfaced ascribing surgical misadventures to "the knife of a tipsy operator." Surgery was a delicate task, and identifying anatomical landmarks, often mangled through combat, was a challenge for a sober surgeon; it was almost impossible when done through eyes blurred by the consumption of too much alcohol. One unfortunate soldier bled to death when "the operator was too drunk to take up the arteries."[41]

In too many cases a hostile disrespect developed between patient and doctor. Military doctors, some of whom were on a zealous search-and-destroy mission for malingering, replaced compassion with callousness, which sometimes fueled a volatile response from openly defiant patients. The emotional explosions were sometimes accelerated by alcohol.

George H. Hood was the acting assistant surgeon at the U.S. Hospital in Westport, Missouri.[42] The hospital was full of activity, and staffing was a constant problem. There were other pressures, such as commanders who wanted troops returned to duty as soon as possible. Perhaps Dr. Hood thought most of the patients were goldbrickers anyway—the sick ward furnishing a respite from the tedium of camp life. Doctor Hood may have privately lamented the swollen sick rolls and decided to obtain relief by purging the bloated census. Among those he deemed medically fit for discharge was Pvt. Lewis Wengartner.

Morning medical rounds were conducted each day. These were brief bedside visits, during which important decisions regarding the disposition of patients were made. Patients eligible for discharge were notified early so preparations could be coordinated for their return to duty. As Dr. Hood approached Wengartner, the acting assistant surgeon perfunctorily announced the patient's imminent discharge. Wengartner protested, defiantly challenging Dr. Hood because he "was totally unfit to perform the duties of a soldier." Dr. Hood did not apparently appreciate this challenge to his military medical authority, and a heated argument stoked passions further; Dr. Hood's anger turned physical.

A surgeon standing trial for assault and battery was a rare occurrence. Dr. Hood argued his case well, and after hearing both sides of the story, the court-martial was decided in his favor. The charge of assault and battery was dismissed, ultimately not considered an offense by court members except when coupled with a proven intent to kill the victim. Lesser charges were similarly disposed of, and Dr. Hood was released back to duty.

Military discipline was expected of patients admitted to hospitals. Uniforms were worn, except when medical practice dictated otherwise. The hospital environment, so different from that of regular duty, might have blurred boundaries between medical officers and patients. An atmosphere of entitlement for care and concern occasionally clouded a patient's judgment, and storms developed when behavior turned malevolent. The hospital provided no shelter from military law.

Admission to the hospital ward transferred the soldier's military duty to that location. Patients were not free to leave without permission. Private Hiram Reed learned that lesson the hard way. Following his admission to the post hospital, Reed took the liberty of embarking on an unauthorized absence to go out and drink some local whiskey. He was promptly charged with one day's AWOL. The hospital steward assigned to Reed's care following his return received a full blast of his patient's fury. "I'll attend you hereafter . . . and you tell the surgeon to shove it." Reed's intemperate conduct cost him a court-martial.[43]

Private Frank Moll was admitted to Lawson General Hospital in St. Louis. If Moll's intent was to avoid further hazardous military duty, he succeeded. Threatening to desert, Moll dramatically "[took] his uniform jacket, and with his knife cut said jacket to pieces, said jacket being the authorized uniform." Moll added fuel to the emotional fire he started by further declaring, "Here goes the Union. . . . Hurrah for Jeff Davis." Alcohol was suspected to be influencing his behavior.

Moll was convicted of conduct to the prejudice of good order and military discipline, and he was sentenced to hard labor for three months, the first seven days of which, bread and water comprised his meager nourishment.[44]

The most casual survey of military life uncovered alcohol's influence: Alcohol was a favorite recreational pursuit, doctors extolled its pharmacological benefits, and commanders used it to motivate troops, since moderate use was considered acceptable. Intemperance, however, was all too common. The dark side of immoderation contributed to madness, malingering, and malfeasance.

Alcohol-related misconduct tested the fairness and open-mindedness of the military legal system. Confounding the reach for equity was a lack of public consensus defining alcohol's role in American life. Social attitudes were mixed, often conflicting with military traditions, which in turn collided with an emerging medical model of alcoholism. The sheer number of alcohol-related misbehaviors in the military forced the legal system into relatively uncharted terrain. Justice demanded that new concepts be considered, old punishments reevaluated, and the role of alcohol reassessed in military life. The Civil War experience did not resolve the complex legal issues, but it did provide a foundation for permitting the introduction of new kinds of evidence.

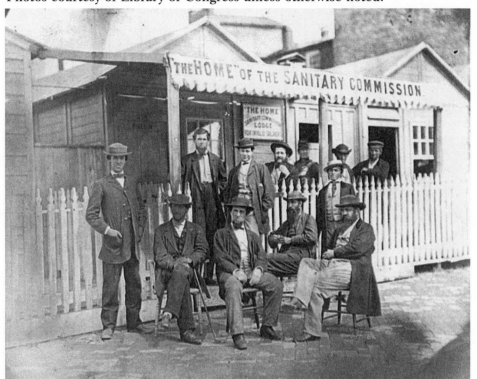

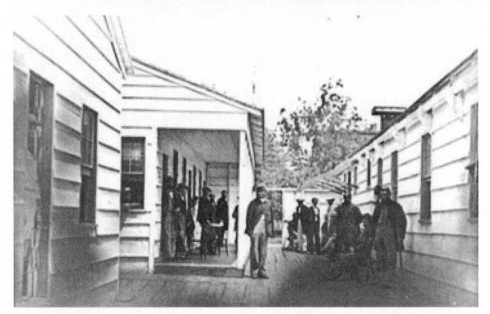

Workers and convalescent soldiers outside the Sanitary Commission's headquarters in Washington, D.C. The commission was a private charity founded early in the war by religious leaders, medical professionals, and concerned citizens with the exclusive mission of monitoring and aiding the health and welfare of soldiers and prisoners of war.

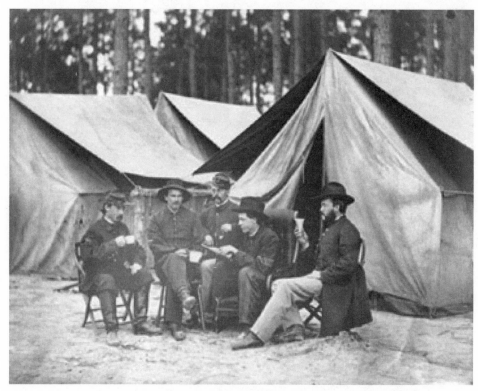

Hospital stewards of the Second Division, Ninth Corps, in front of tents at Petersburg, Virginia. Stewards provided the first line of medical support for soldiers in need

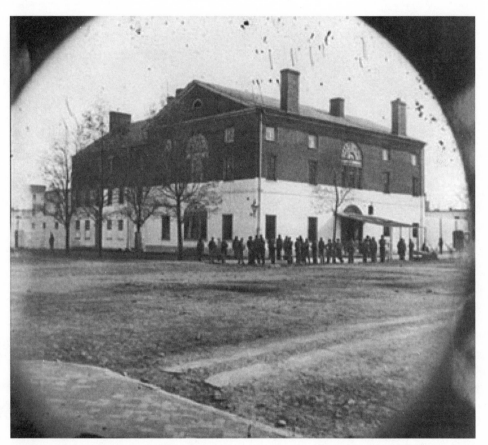

The United States Jail on Washington, D.C.'s Capitol Hill. It had housed the U.S. Congress between 1814 and 1825 after the original Capitol building was burned in the War of 1812, giving rise to the Civil War era name, the Old Capitol Prison. The present-day U.S. Supreme Court was built on the site between 1929 and 1932.

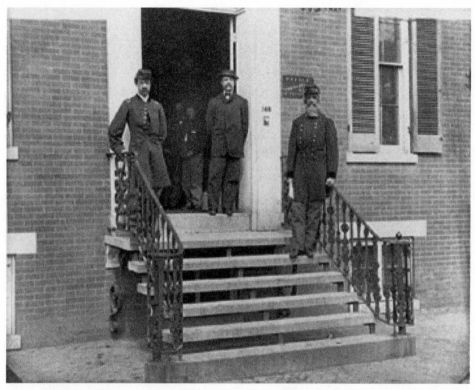

Gen. William Hoffman, the Union Army's commissary general of prisoners (at right) and his staff. Hoffman was responsible for the oversight of both Union and Confederate prisoners.

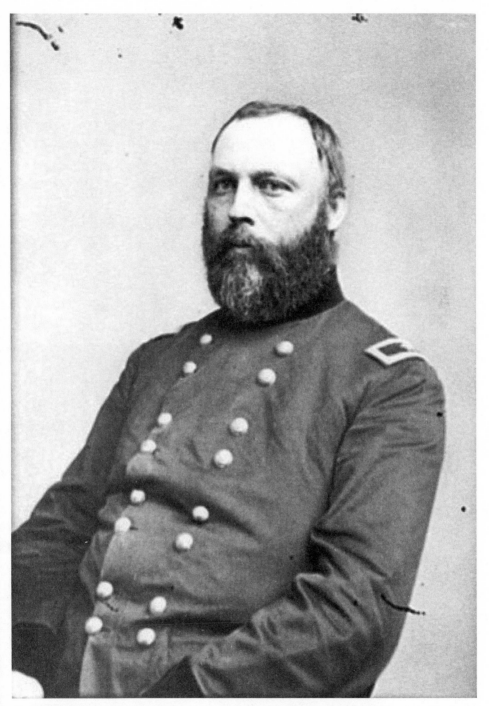

Brig. Gen. William A. Hammond, surgeon-general of the Federal army. Hammond locked horns with Secretary of War Edwin Stanton over the issue of medical incompetence and the organization of the medical department. Hammond was relieved of his position in 1863 and, after demanding a public hearing, court-martialed for mismanagement in a sensational 1864 trial. His controversial medical career continued after the war.

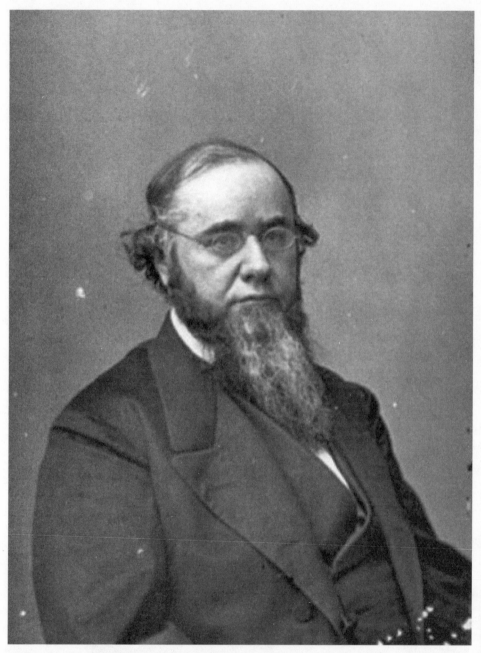

U. S. secretary of war Edwin M. Stanton. Prior to the war in 1859, Stanton argued an early and successful insanity defense that acquitted New York congressman and future brigadier general Daniel Sickles of murder.

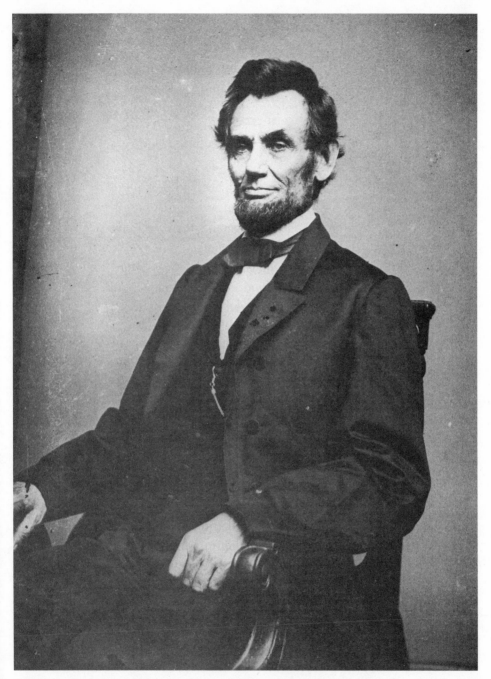

President Abraham Lincoln gained a reputation for compassion towards the common soldier. He personally reviewed hundreds of requests for clemency, including that of Pvt. Leroy Shear, a.k.a. "Lorenzo Stewart." National Archives

CHAPTER FOUR

LIFE IN PRISON

Pretrial confinement was simple. The exigencies of combat required simple, but effective, guardhouses of various types. Depending on the numbers of prisoners to be confined, a tent, barracks, or any building might be used. Court-martial sentences were generally served in the offending soldier's military unit. Extended periods of incarceration were costly, tying up valuable resources, so a serious offense would land a soldier in a local jail or state prison.

Attention during the rebellion focused on housing prisoners of war (POW), and the inundation of prisoners was felt by both sides. In some respects, jailing criminals was easier than incarcerating POWs. Nutrition and sanitation of prisons never suffered the deplorable deprivations associated with the Confederate POW camp at Andersonville, Georgia, or the Union POW camp at Point Lookout, Maryland.

Civilian or military criminals served their sentences in local jails or state prisons, and the large concentration of federal forces surrounding Washington, D.C., strained those local resources. Although authorities scrambled to bolster prison capacity, it was an uphill struggle.

The United States Jail was located on Capitol Hill in the beleaguered Union capital. The facility was dubbed a less ceremonious,
but more descriptive name—the Old Capitol Prison.[1] In the year preceding the war, the United States Jail steadily built a dark reputation.
Inmates and guards alike chafed under strict discipline. Wardens
were empowered to fill and create vacancies as needed, and temporary shortages could be filled with substitutes. Prison regulations
directed that, "If any guard . . . of the prison did not appear for the
purpose of discharging the duties assigned him, that the substitute,
shall receive one half of the pay of such delinquent guard . . . in case
of sickness, and full pay when the party so delinquent is not sick."[2]
The prison could not operate without adequate staffing.

Wall guards were easily the most visible sign of prison security,
and maintaining internal control was one of their essential tasks. A
more subtle, diplomatic mission undertaken by the wall guards was
comforting the civilian populace. Their presence signaled strength
and offered security to a nervous city. Vigilance was the essential
task. Wall guards prevented all but a small contingent of authorized
individuals from ascending the parapets. Another activity the guards
monitored was illicit communication between the convicts and citizens outside the walls. While many such conversations were casual,
satisfying curiosity and relieving boredom, there was a risk in allowing
such communication: Sympathetic listeners might assist escapes.
Accordingly, prison regulations forbade any contact between inmates
and bystanders, and it was wall guards who enforced the rule. Sometimes more than words were exchanged between prisoners and citizens—occasionally, objects would be tossed over the prison walls.
Any such event required the wall guards to submit an immediate
report for the warden's review.

A convict's daily existence at the Old Capitol Prison was a strict,
spartan affair, and initiation to it was sudden and cold, delayed only
briefly by the obligatory diversion to see the prison physician. All
newly assigned inmates underwent a medical examination. Those

found to be in acceptable condition could enjoy the full range of work details.

After the physical exam, the new inmate took a quick bath, and the barber provided a "hair cut close, as prescribed by law." The inmate's civilian clothes were confiscated. Those items judged wearable were stored, while dilapidated clothing was thrown out. Prisoners were not allowed to keep any money, it being considered a contraband item that typically funded illicit commerce. The warden secured all money, issued a receipt, and, upon discharge, returned the funds.

Stripped of his civilian clothing, the convict was made to wear the prison uniform. Distinctive clothing served several purposes: Escape was complicated by the necessity of obtaining civilian clothes, and apprehension was easy when prisoners lacked the foresight to do so. Prison garb was also a constant physical reminder to the convict of his altered status. "The clothing for each convict [was] a rounder about or overjacket, a vest and pantaloons, made of wool for the winter and cotton or linen for the summer, with stripes running round or up and down the body and limbs, a cap of the same cloth, leather shoes and woolen socks, and shirts of coarse cotton or linen."

From April to September the inmates' day began early, around 6:00 A.M., and for the next twelve hours, a variety of work details occupied their time. Convicts were closely monitored. Lollygagging was frowned upon at the first offense and punished on subsequent occasions. Prisoners were expected to be industrious. The twelve-hour grind was relieved on Saturday, when, in deference to the coming Sabbath, the convict's workday concluded in mid-afternoon. Cold weather and diminished daylight, standard features of a Washington winter, demanded a modified work schedule. During this period, inmates left their cells shortly after sunrise and returned at sunset. The relief the prisoners might have felt as a result of the shortened workday was replaced by exasperation at unevenly heated cells.

A bell governed the sleep cycle, and inmates were not allowed to rise from bed or lie down until the signal was given. When they were allowed to sleep, the prisoners likely found the simple arrangements a welcome refuge. "Each convict shall have a mattress, two blankets, made of coarse woolen yarn, not less than one and a half yards wide and two and a half yards long, and one coarse sheet of the same size."

The new inmate was given a stern lecture upon arrival. The rules of the prison were laid out, with obedience constituting the prime directive. Every convict was exhorted to maintain constructive activity, as laziness would result in punishment. Fights, verbal or physical, among jail residents were strictly forbidden. A model prisoner was quiet, anticipated an officer's instructions, and dispatched work duties efficiently. The use of liquor, perhaps the hardest restriction, was also forbidden. One exception permitted liquor when "prescribed by the Physician, when sick in the hospital."

Another restriction, suffered with silent indignation, was the disallowance of tobacco use. As a motivational tool, the warden reserved the privilege of dispensing tobacco for special occasions. The warden might "as a mark of his approbation of their good conduct" reward compliant inmates with a measure of tobacco.

Inmates were expected to observe decorous behavior at all times, and taking a deferential stance toward authority was a wise choice on the part of a prisoner. Noise, whether to express joy, distract, or entertain, brought a certain rebuke. "No convict shall laugh, dance, whistle, sing, run, jump or do anything which will tend to alarm or disturb the prison."

Inmates were compelled to respect jail property, and wanton destruction of the building, furniture, or clothing was not tolerated. Even so, many dwellers in the United States Jail left their mark discreetly. A name, date, and possibly a short lament were etched into a cell's wall. In this small way, the inmates defied a prison rule, while carving out a historical niche for themselves.

Inmates who flaunted institutional orders were punished. They were removed from the general population to solitary confinement and their daily diet was reduced to bread and water. The warden was limited to imposing twenty days confinement for each offense. In some cases, the aggregate number of violations might produce a rather lengthy sentence. A mechanism for mercy existed in the visits made by the Board of Inspectors, preserving at least the appearance of fairness.

A member of the Board of Inspectors conducted weekly site visits, providing an external review of internal operations. In addition to examining the physical structure of the facility, board members had the opportunity to meet with the convicts. It was during these visits that inmates undergoing solitary confinement could make a verbal application for relief, and suitably swayed inspectors might ameliorate the sentence. A less frequent venue for appeal occurred when the Board of Inspectors convened a monthly meeting, where written requests from inmates were reviewed, and at the Board's discretion, might result in a reduction of sentence.

Prison life was calculated to subtract most of life's daily pleasures. A dull, repetitive routine coupled with enforced subservience made up the majority of the convict's experience. The forced institutional dependence was a constant reminder of the prisoner's lost freedom. Among the few distractions brightening the gloom of prison life was the daily diet. Wise wardens understood the role that food played in shaping behavior. Too little or poor quality food caused widespread grumbling, or even rioting, if provisions deteriorated too far. Both the administration and occupants were forever vigilant around this issue: Wardens sought an economical fare, while inmates expected a living portion. An official compromise allowed "12 ounces of pork or 16 ounces of beef; 10 ounces of wheat flour . . . 12 ounces of Indian meal; ½ gill of molasses; and 2 quarts of rye, 4 quarts of salt, 4 quarts of vinegar, 1½ ounces of pepper, and 2½ lbs potatoes, to each hundred rations." This meager diet was later supplemented by tea, sugar, rice, and fish. These luxuries were issued with the admonition that the warden must prudently "support the health and strength of the convicts, having always a proper regard for the economy of the penitentiary."

Every inmate looked forward to release, and when that happy moment arrived, the warden had one last chance to influence the inmate. At a minimum, the warden would inquire about "the means of moral and religious instruction . . . the early temptations to crime to which he was exposed . . . his habits, predominant passions, and prevailing vices." The conversation was recorded in a prison directory, and a certificate of discharge issued. The chastened and possibly rehabilitated inmate was now free to rejoin society.[3]

An awkward relationship sometimes developed between the warden and physician. The warden was principally concerned with security and discipline, and he ruled with almost absolute authority. Physicians were, by nature and training, an independent group, and their control of all things medical sometimes clashed with the warden's goals. The physician could influence work details, transfer an inmate to the infirmary, or comment on the prison's environmental health. Not bound by the prison organizational hierarchy, an aggressively motivated physician could be the proverbial bull in a china shop.

Dr. William H. Duhamel did not shy away from controversy. He took his appointment as physician to the United States Jail seriously. His frequent rounds and ministrations to the ailing inmates afforded him close observation of the jail's shortcomings. In time, Dr. Duhamel grew frustrated, as the special needs of his sick patients were ignored. On one occasion, Duhamel had written an order prescribing wine for a patient; however, the warden, in an open attack on the doctor's authority, silently refused to requisition the item. Perhaps more troubling to the doctor was a lack of food, particularly when sick inmates were being denied their quota.

Dr. Duhamel would not be thwarted without a fight. Bypassing the warden, he pled his case directly to James Harlan, the Secretary of the Interior. "I would respectfully request that instructions be given to the Warden of the Jail to make more definite arrangements concerning the issuance of food to the sick at the jail as on several occasions of late the sick failed to get their rations." Dr. Duhamel was particularly upset and illustrated his complaint by describing an inmate who had received no food for an entire day.[4]

Duhamel maintained a fairly regular correspondence with the Secretary of the Interior. His determined efforts to eradicate an epidemic of typhoid at the prison were well known. For three months,

Dr. Duhamel labored amidst the frightful contagion, and his efforts were largely successful.

In plying his profession, Duhamel remained sensitive to financial prudence, and, through his frugal policy of medical administration, he achieved significant cost savings. Prior to Dr. Duhamel's tenure, prescription costs were approaching five hundred dollars a year, and, without sacrificing patient care, Duhamel was able to whittle in-house prescription costs down to two hundred dollars a year.

Dr. Duhamel was a valuable asset. His principled medical ethics and wise administrative procedures supplemented his genuine compassion for people. Because his benevolence contradicted the warden's goal of punishment, a permanent barrier was erected between the two men. However, despite his differences with the warden, Duhamel managed to maintain a civil working relationship with him. Citing his contributions, Duhamel wrote a letter to the interior secretary requesting an increase in salary from eight hundred to one thousand dollars a year. Three months later, the doctor's contributions were recognized, and he was awarded a pay raise. Without the support of the warden, the pay raise would have been summarily rejected.

Inmates housed at the Old Capitol Prison were a motley crew. Both civilian and military individuals shared space. Men and women, "colored and white," were routinely admitted. Age made little difference. Seasoned older criminals were available to mentor juvenile offenders. The population fluctuated throughout the war, from the low one hundreds to a high of nearly three hundred prisoners. Although the population surged, the physical structure of the prison was unyielding. When the prison was designed, the planners envisioned it housing about one hundred inmates. The jail consisted of twenty-two cells, each measuring eight by ten feet. Additional space consisted of ten rooms, which were designed to hold six occupants each.[5]

Roughly 10 percent of the jail's prisoners were women, some of whom were charged with a variety of offenses, ranging from larceny and assault, to nonpayment of fines. A larger group were detained secondary to "keeping [a] Bawdy-house."[6]

Prison officials eventually recognized the danger of housing youthful offenders (children under the age of sixteen) alongside older inmates. The number of juvenile offenders at the United States Jail was never large. Both boys and girls were incarcerated. There were options for alternate incarceration, but the choices were limited. Juvenile offenders could temporarily be detained at the United States Jail while awaiting placement in a house of refuge, which were located in many major cities, such as Baltimore and Philadelphia.

Juvenile offenders found little to rejoice about when they were transferred from the United States Jail to a house of refuge, where they were still considered prisoners and housed in cells. As they were for their adult counterparts, obedience and silence were mandated for the juveniles as well. In a hopeful attempt to rehabilitate the young prisoners' minds, moral education that borrowed heavily from religion was provided at the houses of refuge. Prisoners who became restless, disenchanted, or mischievous were reminded that "[a]t-tempting to break Jail, is a State Prison offense."[7]

Overcrowding and dilapidation contributed to escape attempts, which were common at the United States Jail. In 1865, the warden of the jail wrote with exasperation that "With all the care and watch-fulness exercised in guarding the prisoners, still it is of frequent occurrence that they are detected in cutting holes through the walls to make their escape. I have found it necessary to iron-clad three of the cells, and otherwise to improve the building to make it more secure."[8]

Convicts that successfully fled the United States Jail were aggressively hunted. Newspapers advertised rewards for the capture of escapees. The value of the reward bore some relationship to the nature of the crime: Five hundred dollars was offered for George W. Johnson. Johnson "convicted of manslaughter and robbery . . . was born in the city of Washington, D. C. where his parents and brothers reside, is a carpenter by trade, has the following hieroglyphics on person, marked with India ink: on right arm, a wreath encircling the letters J. T. J., a small heart and a small circle; . . . [he] has sandy hair, and light eyebrows, is 5 feet 2½ inches high, foot 9⅞ inches long."[9]

Prison records memorialized the inmates who passed their time at the United States Jail.[10] Their foul deeds, big or small, were dutifully inscribed in small logbooks along with their names, charges, and commitment dates. The influence of the war was reflected in charges that might not have been criminal offenses outside of the military environment: Desertion, straggling, drunkenness, and absence without pass were common offenses.

J. G. Biescoe was briefly detained at the Old Capitol Prison, charged with the crime of larceny. When his sentence expired, the warden met with Biescoe just prior to his release. When the warden asked him where he intended to go after his discharge, Biescoe flippantly replied, "Wherever [I] like." Another soldier, C. Flynn, was jailed for robbing a fellow soldier. Upon release, he was returned to his regiment under military guard.

A logbook entry for inmate T. Fuller rather embarrassingly displayed an official ignorance of his release destination. Fuller had been charged with multiple offenses that included forging pay records, desertion, and murder, crimes serious enough to have justified more attention to his eventual whereabouts. Fuller was variously listed as being returned to his regiment, sent to Fort Whipple, Virginia, or Hardwick Hospital. One entry, more honestly perhaps, simply listed his release destination as "unknown."

There was no similar lack of clarity regarding the destination of Henry Weinz, who was convicted of murder. A few months after his release, he was executed in Washington. Likewise, Harvey Brown, an officer in the Kentucky Cavalry, emotionally decompensated during incarceration. He was transferred to the Government Hospital for the Insane.

The Old Capitol Prison served as a transfer point for many inmates, and the crush of admissions forced a feverish hunt for alternate placements. Recipients of the Old Capital Prison's inmates included Ft. Delaware, Delaware; Ft. Whipple, Virginia; Johnson's Island, Ohio; Albany Penitentiary, New York; and Sing Sing State Prison, New York.

The Old Capitol Prison housed mostly military prisoners during the Civil War, and the minority of civilian prisoners incarcerated there had been jailed for committing military-like crimes. The civilian workforce was essential to prosecuting a successful war, and, while their contribution was duly recognized, it was by no means as hazardous as the job performed by members of the military. Sometimes a crosscurrent of suspicions surrounded healthy men who avoided the military. Money, family, and phony medical conditions were sources of corruption at local draft boards. Another concern, amplified by the war, was a person's loyalty. Determination of a civilian's patriotic disposition was complicated by the lack of a military uniform. Freedom from this external symbol made it easier for a person to fraternize with the enemy. A litmus test, in the form of an oath of allegiance, was applied in suspect situations. Any person who failed to swear an oath of allegiance when asked to do so was subject to arrest.

The prison docket recorded one such man, who "say's he's Twenty six years old . . . was arrested on the 11th of August at the Navy Yard Washington where he had been working for some three days . . . was asked to take the Oath and refused. . . . Has been working on railroads and farms in Virginia for the last nine years. Has never done anything for the rebel army. . . . His ignorance got him into trouble. Is perfectly willing to take the Oath. Recommended his Discharge on Oath."[11]

Living in Virginia as a noncombatant naturally suggested a civilian's tendency to favor the Confederacy. Daniel Vowles was scooped up as a rebel sympathizer, in spite of his having made a previous oath of allegiance to the U.S. government. Vowles was a thirty-five-year-old farmer in Fairfax County, Virginia, who plowed his land throughout the war. It was a sparsely populated area, but whispers about Vowles traveled quickly and soon reached the ears of federal authorities. On the strength of innuendo, Vowles was arrested. He was considered "disloyal and . . . a dangerous person to be at large." Daniel Vowles was transported up north to the Old Capitol Prison, no doubt, protesting his innocence. His release was entirely contingent on meeting one demand—that he make another oath. Vowles repeatedly assured his captors that he was "willing to renew his oath."[12]

Other civilians earned their stay at the Old Capitol Prison by more conventional means. War provided crafty entrepreneurs with all sorts of new opportunities to make money or engage in espionage. It was the latter path that J. Veneman trod.

John Scully sent mixed messages. He outwardly manifested an unyielding fidelity to the Union, by donning his country's uniform as a faithful measure of his convictions. A subtle discontent contributed to a more complex, ambiguous picture of Scully. J. Veneman was adept at identifying and exploiting divided loyalties. In his guise as a milk peddler, Veneman had access to military regiments stationed in Washington, D.C., and it was while Veneman was in that role that Scully made his acquaintance. "I purchased milk from him on several occasions and we got intimate. . . . One day he asked me what I was going to fight for. I informed him that I was fighting for the revenge of the death of my two brothers and the loss of my two fingers which I lost for fighting for the Union. . . . He then left and came back the same day and brought me some whiskey. . . . After partaking of the liquor he wished to know of me if I would not like to join another service and receive a large bounty of $400.00 and that he could put me across the river the same night with himself to the Confederate Army."

To his credit, Scully was sufficiently alarmed to inform his superiors of Veneman's offer, and, from that meeting, a plot was hatched to snare the unsuspecting collaborator. Scully arranged to meet with Veneman one more time. Veneman no doubt expected a favorable response to his generous offer, but instead military detectives surprised him and arrested him. After Veneman's arrest, but prior to his trial, Scully was asked by jail officials to identify the conspirator. "I have seen the man and I can testify that he is the same person, only that he has shaved, his whiskers off . . . he is dressed in the same style as he was when he made me the above offer to join the Rebel Army, except that he had on a checkered coat." Veneman may have had some valid doubts about Scully, but, to his detriment, he misjudged the magnitude of Scully's ambivalence. It was that miscalculation that sealed Veneman's fate.[13]

Prisoners incarcerated at the Old Capitol Prison during the war had few diversions. Food and the occasional visitor were among the chief pleasantries punctuating a rather bleak existence. Although inmates were permitted visitors, all visitors were searched for contraband and were required to read and sign the ubiquitous oath of allegiance: "In availing myself of the benefits of this pass I do solemnly swear (or affirm) that I will support, protect, and defend the Constitution and Government of the United States against all enemies, whether domestic or foreign, and that I will bear faith, allegiance, and loyalty to the same, any ordinance, resolution, or law of any state convention or legislature to the contrary notwithstanding; and further, that I do this with full determination, pledge and purpose, without any mental reservation or evasion whatsoever: so help me God."[14] Some visitors might have had to swallow their pride when signing the oath, but the consequence of refusing was obvious.

Rations fluctuated sometimes in response to the warden's benevolence. Those that thought of prison as punishment might use meager rations to further the inmates' pain. Wardens more disposed to a philosophy of rehabilitation carefully weighed the impact of restricted rations on behavioral change. Diets influenced by the more charitable attitude were generally more nutritious. "The rations consist of mackerel, with wheat bread and coffee, for breakfast; beef and cornbread for dinner. Salt fish, bacon, beans, potatoes and soup are also served them on different days, while the sick have rice, tea, molasses, and good wheat bread."[15]

The military anticipated the necessity of secure stockades located outside the nation's capital. Even before the prospect of prisoners of war loomed large, the military properly concluded that traditional criminals would need placement in other facilities. Existing state penal institutions were used for transfers, but this was never an entirely satisfactory solution, because bureaucratic entanglements complicated the transfers, and the military lost all control of the inmates once they were housed in state facilities. Military prisons were essential.

Throughout the war, the military struggled vainly to house vast numbers of prisoners. Most were confused, dispirited prisoners of war, who faced a harsh, often brutal, existence following capture. In part, that inhospitable reception resulted from the crushing volume, which limited resources available to expend on their care, and the lack of consistently applied rules that governed the overall treatment of prisoners of war. Curiously, while never enjoying what would be called a luxurious existence, in some respects, criminals fared better than prisoners of war. Again several factors might have accounted for the difference in treatment, such as the felon's proximity to family, the absence of the enemy label, smaller numbers, and America's greater experience in dealing with criminals as opposed to prisoners of war.

CHAPTER FIVE

MANY FACES OF MALINGERING

Malingering, best defined as the willful fabrication of physical or emotional symptoms to avoid an unwanted duty, was common. The art of playing sick was practiced at all levels. Most soldiers only briefly rehearsed their scenes before going public, but others were polished actors, taking time and care to ensure a flawless performance. Members of these "acting troupes" occasionally provided return engagements. Some were unmasked, but most were not. Unlike stage actors, these military performers were not seeking applause or adulation, their goal was more banal. By depicting the drama of distress, the actor was inspired to fool his audience. Each observer, from messmate to surgeon had to believe the false symptoms were genuine. Failure meant more than a scathing review: Fellow soldiers would hurl a withering rebuke and commanders would punish the wayward performer. Despite the risks of humiliation and disgrace, soldiers were attracted to this version of the limelight.

Soldiers playing the sick role were motivated by greed, but the illusion they presented served to distract others from finding out the truth. If his guise was discovered, however, the malingerer was revealed as a plain coward. Cloaking his identity behind a mask of illness, the malingerer stole social benefits that should have been reserved for the truly disabled. He sought sympathy, safety, and a face-saving exit from military service.

A vast underground network supported malingering, and the weight of patriotism, duty, and honor never collapsed the structure. Resilience was built from basic human emotions such as entitlement, resentment, and fear. Fakers were assisted in the act of deception by quacks, sympathetic physicians, "professional brokers," and family members, whose imprecise knowledge of human pathology some-times offered the key that unlocked the lie.

Adding further support to the underground network was a solid plank of inequity. The ill-conceived option of draft substitution favored the rich. Those with means had a socially sanctioned escape from the unpleasantness of performing military duty. For a tidy sum, a rich man could hire a substitute to take his place in the draft and legitimately relieve him of his obligation. On the surface, this act of commerce among agreeable individuals appeared to be fair, but the inequity lay just below the surface. The perception persisted that this particular social contract benefited the privileged few—at the expense of the less fortunate. Malingering could be conceptualized as the poor man's answer to the practice of draft substitution, although it lacked the social gloss of approval. The ability to successfully feign an illness would insulate the actor from social criticism. After all, who could be faulted for suffering a medical disqualification?

Malingering was expensive, and soldiers who consciously manipu-lated the system left behind a debt. The honest people who remained were held liable, and each paid a portion of the cost through increased exposure to hazardous duty. An undetermined number paid with their lives.

Malingering also took a toll on group cohesion. The scam was often suspected, but rarely punished. When flagrant examples of malingering were ignored, cynicism corroded command authority. When soldiers saw others successfully shirking their responsibilities, they were encouraged to do the same, and at times soldiers' combined ailments threatened to collapse their military units.

Surgeons grew increasingly callous, skeptical, and distrustful of everyone, as malingering spread, causing them to occasionally mislabel legitimate illness as fakery. Honest soldiers became frustrated and resented such accusations. Some seethed with anger, in silence; others expressed their irritation openly, only to earn punishment for their directness. Indirectly, anger was reflected in poor performance or "a bad attitude." To avoid this spectacle, an untold number of soldiers simply didn't see the surgeon, trading the prospect of group derision for physical discomfort. As a result, their untreated illnesses undermined their combat readiness.

Malingering was frequently undertaken in anticipation of some unpleasant event, like an impending battle. Suppressing any apprehension, the soldier coolly and dishonestly paraded his discomfort to comrades, commanders, and the surgeon. Malingering not only violated the moral principle demanding honesty, it breached the military ethic requiring teamwork and individual sacrifice. Group morale depended on accurate detection of malingering, and both commanders and surgeons remained vigilant to detecting such abuses. Between surgeons and soldiers a curious cat and mouse game occasionally developed. Doctors sought to snare soldiers who feigned illness with their own medical deceptions, and to do so, they employed clever diagnostic maneuvers and aggressive, almost sadistic, conventions.

Confirming an episode of malingering was difficult. Generally, the malingerer was more motivated than anyone else. The commander's attention was distracted by the necessities of military life. Overworked surgeons were forced to triage serious injury or illness, their precious time devoted to likely survivors. As a result, mortal cases and minor problems received less medical attention, and these cursory medical exams worked to the advantage of the artful dodger.

Desperation wrote the script for many malingerers. An ache or a cough was insufficiently dramatic, so these misfits enlivened their acts with self-inflicted wounds, guaranteeing at least temporary relief from combat.

Malingering was a military crime involving conscious preparation with the specific intent to avoid performing military duty.[1] The method differed from straggling, skulking, or desertion, and, although the end result of all four methods seemed similar, in actuality, malingering enjoyed a bonus. A successful actor not only avoided some unpleasant activity, but also was rewarded with sympathy. Sickness was the perfect exchange for laziness. This face-saving fraud spared the malingerer the harsher sobriquet of cowardice.

From the standpoint of moral culpability, malingering usually weighed less than desertion. The goal of skulking, straggling, and desertion was obvious, meriting major disdain. Curiously, the fusing of criminal intent with medical symptoms softened the cry for punishment. In some respects, malingering was even more odious than cowardice, the long planning and the stealing of sympathy arguing for harsher punishment. Most malingerers feigned symptoms that were subjective, challenging the surgeon's diagnostic skill. Prosecution was impossible without the medical evidence to disprove the actor's claim.

Malingering was generally seen on several stages. The actor might present his play during recruitment, during active service, or while he was hospitalized. Conscription bred malingering. Subtracting the highly motivated citizens who had originally volunteered for military service left an undistinguished crowd consisting of two broad types: those who accepted the call to arms with varying degrees of ambivalence, but performed well, and others who were bound and determined to sneak away.[2]

Medical disqualification was a popular way to avoid active service. Physicians were charged with identifying medical disabilities. A fit fighting force depended on healthy recruits, so weeding out infirmity was fundamental. Unfortunately, the system was riddled with abuse. Many civilian physicians, motivated either by compassion or compensation, actively undermined conscription and wrote medical affidavits documenting bogus disabilities. A New York surgeon lamented, "To the disgrace of the profession I am pained to confess that many physicians of high standing both in the profession and the community, either from excessive cleverness or for a consideration, lent them-selves to this disreputable practice." A military surgeon was more dip-lomatic in expressing his disdain. After seeing countless examples of falsified ailments, the surgeon charitably felt that his colleagues, "Per-haps unwittingly," contributed to the practice.[3]

Complicating the honest physician's life were a maze of military regulations. Medical induction criteria were designed to eliminate the physically unfit recruit. Although the intent of the regulations was to guide the selection process, many physicians swore the rules had the opposite effect.

Poorly crafted medical disability policies created more confusion than clarification. Epilepsy was an example. Recognizing a potential for abuse, military regulations declared, "For this disability the state-ment of the drafted man is insufficient, and the fact must be estab-lished by the duly attested affidavit of a physician of good standing who had attended him in a convulsion."[4]

The episodic nature of seizures conspired to undermine this regu-lation. Rarely, would an epileptic have the good fortune to time his seizure for purposes of medical observation. Physicians were baffled. No doubt many provided the necessary documentation based on a commonsense approach—they accepted the validity of a credible his-tory. Other doctors stuck to a literal interpretation of the policy. Fail-ing to observe a seizure firsthand, these physicians would not lend their written authority to a recruit. Consequently, many soldiers with bona fide seizure disorders were inducted, creating the following sce-nario: The sick soldier was sent to a military commander desperately in need of personnel reinforcements. The soldier had a dramatic sei-zure, which scared everyone and forced the soldier's exodus, leaving the commander short one man. It was a costly approach, which vio-lated the very aim of the regulation.

A more disturbing, even ludicrous, medical standard involved nearsightedness. Military regulations explicitly turned a "blind eye" to diminished visual acuity. The implications for inducting a myopic recruit were almost comical. As one surgeon caustically noted, "of what use can a man be to his country, as a soldier, who is unable to discern friend from foe at the usual distance of normal vision?"[5]

Incomprehensible medical recruitment standards were written by bureaucrats who were saddled with various constraints. The need for manpower was the main concern. If there were too many exemptions, there would be a flood of discharges. Some infirmities, for example, feeble vision, were just too common among the populace, and to officially sanction this condition as a medical disability would fundamentally threaten the military's personnel acquisition efforts. The remedy was simple; myopia would not be recognized as a qualifying medical exemption.

Incredibly, military regulations exempted the toothless. Americans suffered from incredibly poor dental health. What started as a few decaying teeth invariably led to a wholesale loss of teeth, although the damage was more cosmetic than functional. Despite the absence of teeth, nutrition was rarely compromised. Large strapping youths, whose only malady was a mouth without teeth, dutifully presented themselves to enrollment board physicians, only to be turned away.

The first written rendition barred entry when a "loss of sufficient number of teeth to prevent proper mastication of food and tearing the cartridge" exists. A subsequent clarification allowed "total loss of all front teeth, the eyeteeth, and first molars even if only of one jaw."[6] The lack of a correlation between dental health and nutritional status made this broad exemption appear inconsistent. Perhaps military planners focused on the rough fare soldiers would have to eat; eating hardtack required good strong teeth.

Carefully crafted medical enrollment standards sought to identify false medical claims. Obvious physical deformities, such as hernias and tooth loss, were not easy to simulate, but rheumatism, heart disease, and various neurological disorders were easily faked. As a result, military regulations demanded greater scrutiny of these illnesses. Instructions to physicians were, in these areas, more detailed in an effort to ferret out malingerers. Rheumatism was a common culprit.

Rheumatism was a term applied to a constellation of subjective

symptoms. All manner of joint and muscle discomforts and vague
bone pains were clumped together under the heading of rheumatism.
When soldiers consciously constructed the symptoms to deceive the
viewer, only the most ardent or accidental observations could uncover
a rheumatic dodger.

"After the battle of Fredericksburg a soldier . . . whose courage
had evidently been put to a sore test . . . resorted to the rheumatic
dodge to secure his discharge. He responded daily to sick call, piti-
fully warped out of shape, was prescribed for, but all to no avail. One
leg was drawn up so that, apparently, he could not use it, and groans
. . . of excruciating agony escaped him at studied intervals and on
suitable occasions."[7] The dodger was consistent in his guise for many
weeks, ultimately resulting in the ultimate reward—a stamp of medical disqualification. Discharge papers were dutifully drawn up and
submitted, and approval was granted through division headquarters.
Final discharge authority was vested in the Army Corps Headquarters, but, in this case, the dodger's deception was discovered as a
result of his carelessness.

Prematurely celebrating his assumed victory, the rheumatic
dodger secured a cask of whiskey, which he shared freely with his
hoodwinked friends. "Not being a temperance man, the dodger was
thrown off his guard by this spiritual bonanza, and, taking his turn at
the straw, for which entry had been made into the barrel, he was soon
as sprightly on both legs as ever. In this condition his colonel found
him."[8] The dodger fell rapidly from his euphoric orbit, was forcefully
grounded, and reinstated in the military.

Feigning rheumatism was a favorite scam among many "volunteers," because the disease was easy to fabricate. In Pennsylvania's
11th District, rheumatism quickly topped the list of ailments from
which inductees suffered. The epidemic was controlled by a decidedly nonmedical prescription: The enrollment board simply refused
to recognize further cases.[9]

If left unchecked, the "scourge" of rheumatism claims could seriously impair combat readiness. Few regiments were entirely immune
to the scam, so, after two years of national struggle, the Union Army

declared war on rheumatism, via command directives ordering the malady into nonexistence. But rheumatism stubbornly refused to be rubbed out.

Military enrollment boards supervised recruitment. Board members could count on draftees to exaggerate the poor status of their health, since the normal objective was to avoid conscription. In some paradoxical cases, the prospective soldier concealed a true disability. While some were motivated by patriotism, others were inspired by greed. Hiding a disability allowed a soldier to capture a recruitment bonus. As soon as he was inducted, the soldier would disclose the physical ailment, causing him to be disqualified from active duty and discharged. Many soldiers repeated this cycle several times, which was a silent indictment of the physical examination procedures.

Enrollment boards were presented with a seemingly endless array of phony conditions. Use of the plant belladonna imitated blindness by dilating the pupils. During the physical examination, the doctor would encounter the fixed, unresponsive pupils. It was a common ruse, but most of these "blind" soldiers were ignorant of the diagnostic implications of their simulation. Fixed pupils signaled a serious neurological problem, such as a prior stroke or brain tumor, which created other deficits like gait abnormalities or limb weakness. When a young person came sashaying in for a physical examination, encumbered only with dilated pupils, the doctor was immediately suspicious.[10]

No discomfort seemed great enough to deter some malingerers. Open sores were sported by the truly fearless. These wounds offered graphic evidence of medical unfitness. An astute surgeon detected the following example.

Nicholas Wee, a melancholy recruit from Minnesota's 2nd District, hobbled in to see the surgeon, sporting painful blisters on both feet. The surgeon didn't reveal what tipped him off. Perhaps it was the fact that the blisters were on both feet, or maybe the recruit appeared to be too cheerful. Maybe the injury just looked contrived. In any event, suspecting his patient of fraud, the surgeon shifted from doctor to detective. The hapless recruit's dreams seemed to come true when the surgeon made arrangements to send him back home. The soldier was gone, but not forgotten. Making a mental note of the case, the surgeon waited two months before springing his trap. After two months, the soldier would no doubt be resting comfortably at home, visions of military life fading from his memory. The soldier was arrested and the surgeon was fully vindicated when no trace of the former injury remained. Through unidentified inducements the recruit confessed to having soaked his feet in lye.[11]

One inventive soldier, from Michigan's 5th District, easily passed his enrollment physical. His next assignment was the general rendezvous, the staging point for subsequent training and transfer. While the soldier awaited transfer, large, ugly sores opened up on both of his legs, and developed a pussy drainage. A surgeon arrived at the obvious conclusion—that the neophyte soldier was unfit for military service and deserved a medical discharge. The military was a small community. Alerted to news of the soldier's imminent discharge, the enrollment board surgeon pressed for further details. The soldier was interrogated and what unfolded was a grand tale of malevolent ingenuity. There was a touch of pride in the soldier's revelation. He had, after all, fooled many folks. Refusing to disclose the exact number, the audacious soldier admitted having enlisted many times. He passed each entrance physical easily and pocketed a fat enlistment bonus. Soon thereafter, painful leg boils mysteriously popped up. Surgeons could never quite figure out the cause or the cure of the boils. The only remedy left was a medical discharge. Unbeknownst to a cadre of surgeons was the fictitious origin of the injury: The soldier had applied a tried and true blistering compound to his legs. The blisters always healed in short order, but by that time, the soldier had already been released from duty. The soldier got rich through the recycling scheme by collecting ill-gotten bounties.[12]

Malingering and masochism every so often were intertwined. The self-inflicted injuries suffered by these soldiers seemed overly destructive, perhaps, in part, reflecting an intense underlying mental distress. Two examples of this curious fusion involved the simulation of emphysema.

A pair of frantic recruits in Minnesota unquestionably wanted out of the Army, and they sought the services of a quack practitioner. Apparently, the physician knew enough about anatomy and disease to perpetuate a hoax. In a painful procedure, the doctor inserted air into the willing victims' lungs through small chest wall punctures. The recruits ran the significant risk of complete lung collapse or a galloping infection. It was unlikely that either party was aware of the risk, because otherwise, they would likely have been deterred from the fraud. One of the two successfully failed his physical and was dismissed, but the other soldier was less fortunate. His ruse was detected and he was inducted.[13]

Military physicians encountered a scourge of wholesale fraud everywhere: by recruits, active duty members, and even hospitalized patients. Grimly determined to defeat the cowardly practice of malingering, military surgeons coached each other on a variety of uncovering techniques. Successful suggestions borrowed on the premise that malingerers were basically a fearful lot. Most malingerers carefully balanced symptoms and pain. The goal was to achieve discharge without a permanent disability or suffering too much discomfort. The perceptive military surgeon could manipulate the malingerer's carefully crafted cost-benefit behavior. The cautious malingerer was forced into disarray when the surgeon escalated the cost of continuing the deception, by, for example, prolonging the period of observation. Facing the greater threat of exposure, many malingerers recalculated their odds and capitulated.

The discovery of chloroform was a boon to humane surgical practice.[14] Although it was slowly added to hospital pharmacies, widespread distribution was affected by national priorities. Weapons were favored over medicines. Even when chloroform was available, attitudes were an obstacle in its easy acquisition. As is the case with any new, mysterious product, fear and myth accompanied its introduction. Shrewd surgeons soon discovered that chloroform had a beneficial side effect. The mystique of chloroform frightened soldiers—and most definitely unnerved malingerers.

Soldiers suspected of malingering were offered a "cure" with a miracle medicine. A draftee from Ohio had his stiff, aching back entirely relieved as he ran from the threat of chloroform. Another draftee from Missouri pathetically limped around the camp, claiming his left knee was stiff and unbending. At sick call the surgeon examined the knee and was unimpressed with the physical findings. Pondering the possibility of a sham, the surgeon retrieved a bottle prominently labeled chloroform. Perhaps the soldier was unaware of chloroform or simply willing to gamble on the outcome. The surgeon administered a sub-anesthetic dose of chloroform. Dazed and confused by the intoxicant, the soldier retained just enough cognition to further the deception. Urging caution, the surgeon asked the soldier to demonstrate his gait. False confidence moved the soldier as he overplayed the part. His right knee appeared even less flexible now. The dismayed surgeon was on the verge of declaring his experiment a failure when a recollection restored his faith. It was the left knee— not the right—that had brought the soldier to sick call. This actor badly bungled his encore performance.[15]

Perhaps malingering was less common among officers. They calculated rather quickly that they simply had more to lose; the benefits of authority softened the rougher edges of military life, and promotion offered the promise of even greater insulation. Once in a while, officers gambled with those advantages, tarnishing both their reputation and that of the military.[16] A case in point involved Lt. Col. Chapman J. Stuart, 14th West Virginia. His performance was unveiled for the exclusive viewing of a military examination board.

The U.S. Congress established military examination boards in 1861, empowering them "to examine the capacity, qualifications, propriety of conduct, and efficiency of any commissioned officer."[17] Too many officers were appointed based on political patronage rather than military experience. While this satisfied the ambitious yearnings of well-connected men, it often came at the expense of good leadership. Unit cohesion and combat victories were hampered by the lack of skill of these popinjay commanders. The Union Army acknowledged the problem, and established military examination boards to measure

the competency of prospective leaders. In theory, every aspiring officer was tested on the basic tenants of warfare.

Military examination boards served another function.[18] They evaluated complaints lodged against commissioned officers. Few mecha-
nisms existed to penetrate the cloistered ranks. Visionaries understood that the military-political wall protecting incompetent officers
ultimately undermined command authority, and without a credible
approach to weed out bad officers, the entire corps was tarnished.
Restoring respect and officer accountability was the foremost consideration when the charter regulations of the military examination
boards were drafted. As evidence of that commitment, the authors
incorporated a mechanism to investigate complaints against officers.
The military examination board functioned in a quasi-judicial
manner.[19]

Limited oversight and broad power offered opportunities for both
efficiency and abuse. When complaints arose, the boards offered a
streamlined approach to justice when compared with the convoluted
court-martial process. Negligent commanders could be administra-
tively, not judicially, removed.

Officer selection was the other role managed by military examination boards, and they exerted both direct and indirect control over the
process. Direct control flowed from the actual examination, but the
boards also exercised an intangible, indirect influence, by causing
some candidates, who were mindful of their deficiencies, to forgo
commissioning altogether. Public humiliation in front of military
authorities, some of whom may have been friends or political opponents, was too great of a potential embarrassment.

Numerous examples of abuse subtracted from the reputation of
the military examination boards. Political patronage, favoritism, and a
raw lust for power infiltrated the dealings of many boards. Commanders might convene a commission expressly to install cronies. Abusing
the board mandate as a sort of administrative Trojan horse, the guile-
ful commander stealthily replaced his subordinates. Experienced
officers were discharged after failing rigged examinations.

Candidates ordered to appear before an examination board, in reality, generally had little to fear. The president of the board prepared the examination; there were no standardized testing formats. The board's whim, and testimonial statements submitted by the candidate, determined the outcome. The range of examinations was broad, with some officers facing hours of grueling questions and others receiving summary judgment after one question. Inquiries focused on the candidate's knowledge of tactics and military regulations. Despite the appearance of rigor, most officers easily passed.

The benign reality of most examination boards was clouded by a shadowy perception. Secret deliberations, subjective grading, and no mechanism for formal appeal cast doubt on the boards' integrity.

Lieutenant Colonel Stuart was acutely aware of the rumors swirling around about the military examination boards. Along with some fellow officers, he was called before a military examination board. Stuart apparently greeted the order with a mixture of rage and panic. Perhaps he considered himself above reproach and was offended by the request, or, on the other hand, he might have feared a public exposé of his ignorance. In any event, Stuart responded to the military examination board with a campaign of political shenanigans, shamming, and a protracted power struggle.

Stuart's first response to the examination order was to dash off a letter to the board president. The letter was poorly conceived, anxiously written, and hastily delivered. A touch of despair permeated the letter, with Stuart claiming illness and seeking a few days delay. Stuart assured the board that a few days convalescence would ensure his full recovery. The postponement was well used to reinforce his precarious position. Stuart apparently reasoned that if delay did not defeat the board, then political intimidation might. In a subsequent communication to the board, the officer made veiled references to the governor of West Virginia, hinting that the governor was considering his imminent promotion to a full colonelcy. Almost too casually, Stuart promised to send the governor's letters to the board. In exchange, Stuart asked the board to submit the results of his examination to the governor. It was a clever attempt at intimidation. The implication was clear; the board risked the governor's wrath if Stuart failed his military proficiency examination.

The board members bristled at Stuart's clumsy interference, and his ham-handed attempt to cow them backfired. The board president fired a volley in return. Demanding Stuart's presence, the board president telegraphed his displeasure to the regimental commander. Stuart suffered a double disgrace: His malingering was publicly disclosed, and he was forced to undergo the competency examination.

The military examination board eagerly awaited Stuart's arrival. For almost a day and a half a relentless interrogation pummeled the artless officer. With Stuart's political maneuvering and malingering fresh in their minds, board members relished the opportunity to humiliate him. The board's disdain was not spent when the examination was concluded. A flawless performance probably would not have convinced the board—and Stuart fell far short of excellence. Instead of rendering judgment, the board recommended retesting in one month. Like a cat playing with its prey, the board's ultimate revenge seemed to be a sadistic waiting game. Stuart remained in a fretful limbo with a figurative Sword of Damocles hanging over his career. The prospect of reexamination was too daunting a notion for Stuart, and, quietly conceding his defeat, he sought and received a military discharge.[20]

America's Civil War created a new casualty. Brave soldiers, enduring months of service, gradually felt themselves rusting. Even the best-tempered steel loses its shine following long exposure to the elements. A handsome patina covers the surface. Generally only brilliance, not function, is lost. But in some cases, perhaps reflecting intrinsic defects in the metal, the damage goes deeper.

Many soldiers lost their emotional vitality, their sharpness having been dulled by months of military service. The emotional patina was rough and raw. Vicissitudes once dismissed were now absorbed. Soldiers' spirits grew heavy, as humor was replaced by pessimism. Decisiveness was destroyed by doubt, and timidity conquered the soul. The weight of military life then fractured these rusted iron-men.

"Excitement, exhaustion, hard work, and loss of sleep broke down great numbers of men who had received no wounds in battle." Indicting himself with this declaration, a despondent officer sought refuge by clinging to a fragment of reason. Fatigue and desperation had created an emotional whirlpool drowning his rationality. Clutching wildly for support, this officer jumped aboard a mental life raft. It was a rickety structure, consciously fabricated from false symptoms. This was a socially dangerous trip but apparently worth the risk to bridge the gap of mental collapse. The officer trod a delicate balance. He had to make himself sick, but not violently so. After some thought and reflection, a potion "of powdered slate pencils in vinegar" was concocted. This officer's story was recalled by Colonel Dawes, of the 6th Wisconsin, as one he had heard during his tenure on a military examination board. The effect of consuming this noxious solution was not recorded; however, the circumstances do suggest that officers could be just as reckless as their subordinates.[21]

The emotion that drove malingering often demanded dramatic behavior. Some particularly desperate characters calculated that a self-inflicted injury guaranteed an exit visa, and, initially, it worked. Soldiers quickly discovered that self-amputated fingers or toes worked best. The general method of choice was to shoot the digits off with a rifle or handgun. A well-executed plan left observers convinced that the injury was accidental or—even better—inflicted during combat. No doubt, many legitimate injuries stirred whispers.

A gruesome scene witnessed during a routine encampment preyed on the mind of Pvt. John D. Billings. Chopping wood was a necessary chore, and pinning the log underfoot was the common practice of securing the log. Whether through fatigue, poor aim, or by design, the ax missed the log but not the boot. Unfazed by his misfortune, the victim, witnessed by Billings, simply removed his boot and, casually, as if he was dumping some offending stone, he upturned the boot and several toes tumbled out of it. The witness to this amazing tableau pursued the story no further. No doubt the soldier hobbled over to the surgeon, who perhaps consoled his suffering with a medical discharge.[22]

Sam Cobb, a private in the 61st Illinois Infantry, was branded for life following a momentary indiscretion—and his feeble attempt to cover it up. The first time Cobb spotted Johnny Reb, "he broke from the ranks and ran, and never showed up until . . . some days later. He then had one of his hands tied up, and claimed that he had been wounded in the fight. The nature of the wound was simply a neat little puncture, evidently made by a pointed instrument, in the ball of the forefinger . . . not a shot had been fired at us." Captain Reddish, Cobb's commander, accused him of a shameless act of self-mutilation. At the end of his military service, "on returning to his old home, he found that his reputation in the army preceded him." Despite moving a considerable distance to the west, Cobb was never able to escape his past.[23]

The extent of self-injury seemed to rise and fall with the fortunes of war. With quick victory eluding either side, the human cost of continuing the war escalated. Duty, honor, and religious beliefs were the personal values that psychologically insulated the soldier, but the reality of war assaulted these values.[24] Desertions, malingering, and crime peaked as group morale foundered. Letters from family usually buoyed the spirits. Effective letter writing was candid and sentimental when both parties exchanged tender thoughts. Soldiers were allowed to complain, cry, or otherwise use the pen as a means of catharsis, and families were expected to absorb and replenish their sons through soothing, supportive, emotional emollients. Sometimes these rules were turned upside down, and instead of supporting the soldier's situation, families encouraged misconduct.

One Connecticut soldier, Henry H. Thompson, sought a consoling, albeit distant, embrace from his wife, but instead, he got a cold shoulder. Letters from his wife were of an incessant whining nature. "I dont think it will be half as much disgrace to you to have you come home as it will be to stay . . . dont stay for . . . a minute nor an hour if you see a chance." To his credit, this particular Connecticut soldier was not lured by his wife's seduction, but others were not so strong.[25]

A New Jersey soldier responded angrily to his wife's silence, and to break the silence, he challenged her fidelity, in that way, probably hoping to provoke a response. The ploy worked, but it did little to cool his hot temper. His wife's response was ambiguous, claiming faithfulness, but seeking permission to "socialize." This destabilizing response festered in the soldier's mind.

Pessimism and paranoia nagged at the soldier. Powerful forces now conspired to pry him loose from the military: Dissatisfaction with the military pushed, and his wife's provocative behavior pulled, and, although he might have thought about desertion, he ultimately chose deception as his way out of the military.

"I want to get out of this thing some way if I can," the soldier wrote his disaffected wife. "I will have to work some plan to get my discharge. I have been stuffing medicine in myself since I been out here. I have been taking Pulsotil, Bryvina, Beladonna, Acoute, Nuy Pom . . . when you write I wish you would send me some Arsnic or some other kind of stuff so as to make me look pale . . . find out at the druggist what will make you look pale and sickly." The soldier's ill appearance was rewarded with a furlough, and his trip home restored the soldier's confidence, reduced his suspicions, and allowed him to complete his tour of duty.[26]

Malingering was like a game. Each participant made moves designed to deceive their opponent. Soldiers donned various disguises, while surgeons parried those moves. Boasting rights went to the victor, and malingerers were certainly not bashful in bringing their deceptions all the way to the physician's backyard—the hospital. Exaggeration extended the hospital stay of many soldiers recovering from a legitimate wound or illness. Time worked to the advantage of the soldier, since prolonged absences from a military unit reduced the probability of return. Having paid their patriotic duty in blood, many soldiers figured a medical discharge was justly due, and some sympathetic surgeons agreed.

A number of factors conspired to inhibit the return of hospitalized soldiers, not the least of which was self-interest. Understaffed hospitals eagerly petitioned for manpower. When military authorities turned a deaf ear to such pleas, medical officers played their trump card. They had wards full of eager patients who were willing to trade combat for hospital service.[27]

Hospitals and their directors enjoyed an unprecedented degree of freedom relative to their field unit counterparts. The medical staff ruled supreme, answering only to the Surgeon General. Field commanders found it difficult to penetrate these medical fiefdoms. From the commander's vantage point, hospitals only admitted patients, even though it might have seemed as if patients never returned to a combat assignment. This was true, particularly when soldiers were evacuated to state hospitals near their homes. In these instances, the far away sounds of battle colluded with homesickness to weaken the bonds of duty, and families mobilized to thwart their son's return to a hostile environment. Considerate state hospital employees joined forces with the soldier-family dyad. It was a surefire formula to limit the number of soldiers who returned to combat.

Patriotic physicians squarely confronted malingering. Having had extensive clinical experience, they were able to make astute observations and comparisons of cases, and some published their findings in medical journals.

Dr. E. P. Buckner from Kentucky's 6th District counseled his colleagues on the perils of malingering by advising physicians to "be absolutely incredulous . . . cautious, watchful, sharp, shrewd, cunning, and quick . . . otherwise he will or can do the government no good . . . and be nothing but a mere top, whirled at the will and by the dexterity of every unfit recruit, sound drafted man, and rascally substitute. Besides these intellectual and moral qualities, the surgeon must have a competent knowledge of anatomy, physiology, and pathology, or he will grope in the dark."[28]

Dr. J. M. Da Costa was a model medical investigator. His interest in clinical research attracted him to a military hospital in Philadelphia, where he studied patients suffering from a vague cardiac disability that he dubbed the "irritable heart." Chief features of the disorder were palpitations, fatigue, and shortness of breath, symptoms that were tailor-made for abuse. Dr. Da Costa seemed to appreciate the disease's potential for fabrication. "It is impossible to discuss any malady to which soldiers are liable without discussing its being feigned. And a malingerer, as is well known, may keep up a rapid action of the heart by a tight bandage around the upper part of the abdomen and lower part of the chest. But, excepting if this be done, the imitation is a very clumsy one. The impostor knows nothing of the character of the cardiac pain. Further making him lie down after undressing causes the heart to return to its natural beat; and then on resuming the erect position, or walking around quietly, it will not, as an irritable heart does, regain its former frequency or irregular rhythm." Da Costa was confident that the "peculiar physical signs of the irritable organ . . . are traits which cannot be copied."[29]

Dr. Da Costa's trivializing dismissal of malingerers was short-sighted. He formed his opinion based on two hundred cases, a small fraction of the soldiers with cardiac complaints. Most had been discovered or discharged long before reaching Da Costa, and without analyzing this larger group, he couldn't make a reliable estimate of malingered heart problems. Basing his prescribed course of treatment on only two hundred cases also cast doubt on the efficacy of his over-all treatment regime for irritable heart. Nonetheless, Da Costa recommended rest as the principal ingredient, benefiting equally organic disease and the leisure-loving loafer.

William Fuller, a Second Assistant Surgeon of the 1st Michigan Infantry Regiment, openly expressed his disgust with malingerers in the most caustic terms. Fuller bitterly complained that, "there is not a village in the land that does not contain discharged soldiers, who make no concealment of their victories over the surgeons."[30] His front line duty managing the diverse ailments presented by hardened soldiers offered a perspective different from the erudite Dr. Da Costa.

Da Costa was the consummate academic, whereas Fuller was the typical workhorse clinician. To Fuller, sick call was a detailed panorama adorned with colorful symptoms, and, like a discerning art critic, it was the surgeon's responsibility to detect fraudulent works. Unfortunately, some medical officers were blinded by ineptitude or politics. Some lost sight of their boundaries and blurred military obligations with a misguided fraternization. "The desire of medical officers to be popular among the men, has no doubt increased the amount of this vice, while it has not added in the least to the popularity of such officers, but has had the reverse effect among all good and true soldiers."[31]

Fuller advocated a combination of medical skill and suspicion in detecting malingering. By developing multiple lines of communication within the regiment, a surgeon could, "[gain] knowledge and information from whatever source it may come, as long as it is consistent with honor."[32]

Fuller was committed to rooting out malingering. In addition to honing his clinical accuracy, he pursued the medical literature for hints, and from these, he harvested eight principles for diagnosing malingering.

> 1st. The appreciation of the moral situation of the subject, and the motives which influence him to simulate, dissimulate or provoke the malady of which he pretends himself to be victim.
>
> 2nd. Comparison of the malady with the age, temperament and mode of life of the individual.
>
> 3rd. The attentive examination of the affected part, the local symptoms which they present, and the impediments to the exercise of function which result from such lesion, or which are attributed to them.
>
> 4th. Careful comparison of these lesions with the development, the color and the general distortion of the organism.
>
> 5th. Study of the cause to which the lesion real, or pretended is attributed.
>
> 6th. Methodical questioning of the subject of the circumstances which accompanied the development of the disease, to the sensation, to the pains, to the hindrance of function thereby produced.
>
> 7th. Proper employment of therapeutic measures, suggested by the morbid state, and the observation of their effects.
>
> 8th. Appropriate excitation to distract the attention of the man, whilst the affected parts are examined or made to move.[33]

Fuller paid a respectful homage to these rules. Commonly feigned conditions, such as blindness, dumbness, or deafness might yield to such analysis rather easily; however, the fabrication of some disorders resisted simple detection and required additional measures. Fuller observed that "diseases of the kidneys are very popular with these shirks and they are very persistent in their assertions of the reality of their disease and any amount of cupping and blistering will not make them own to the contrary. I had one man under my care who was suffering from feigned weak back, and complained of passing enormous quantities of urine, but upon keeping him in one day and having him pass his water in an vessel, I found it to be light color and quite freely diluted with water, considerable quantity of which he had in the vessel before detection."[34]

Fuller's sanguine comments might have influenced Dr. Da Costa had the two ever conversed. As a student of soldiers' knavery, Fuller was impressed with their resourcefulness. "Diseases of the heart have been a great source for getting out of the service and at one time about all a man had to do was to say that he had heart disease and figured his cards a little and he would gain the end desired."[35]

The battle against malingering could not succeed solely through medical efforts, because too many physicians in that effort, wittingly or otherwise, conspired with the malingerer. Reinforcements, in the form of military law, joined medicine in an attempt to counter the internal scourge.

The earliest reference obliquely criminalizing malingering is found in the 1775 American Articles of War. Buried in a section of "additional articles" enacted in November of that year is a prohibition directed against officers. "In all cases where a commissioned officer is cashiered for cowardice or fraud, it be added in the punishment, that the crime, name, place of abode, and punishment of the delinquent be published in the newspapers, in and about the camp, and of that colony from which the offender come, or usually resides; after which it shall be deemed scandalous in any officer to associate with him."[36] The 1775 Articles of War anticipated medical complicity. "[E]very surgeon or mate, convicted of signing a false certificate, relating to the health or sickness of those under his care, shall be cashiered."[37]

Although the evolution of military law in the years preceding the Civil War failed to produce a specific law criminalizing malingering, that did not prevent resourceful prosecution of the behavior. The few cases presented for court-martial were tried under the 62nd Article of War, a catchall specification outlawing conduct that was "to the prejudice of good order and military discipline." The vague construction of the 62nd Article admitted a wide range of disparate offenses. Caught within the net of the 62nd Article were destabilizing behaviors such as gambling, failure to appear as summoned before a court-martial, presenting drunk to a court-martial, shenanigans committed during target practice, inattention to a military school instructor, improperly formulated drug prescriptions, impersonating an officer, mistreatment of a horse, and malingering or self-maiming.[38]

The lax boundary of the 62nd Article simply held that "a crime, therefore, to be cognizable by a court-martial . . . must have been committed under such circumstances as to have directly offended against the government and discipline."[39] It was a convenient definition that allowed prosecution of unusual crimes without invoking a statutory requirement to amend the military code.

Capt. Alfred O. Brooks was an officer assigned to the 29th Regiment of Massachusetts Volunteers. The reality of war had quickly stripped Captain Brooks of any romantic sentiments of achieving glory on the battlefield. Military life was not only difficult, it was dangerous. There were enjoyable aspects of an officer's life, such as the seemingly endless social engagements. Frustrating Brooks's pursuit of a gentlemanly life was that nagging military obligation, so he searched for a means to retain the prestigious benefits of the uniform, without keeping the burdensome responsibility. Captain Brooks eventually settled on cooking up some fake complaints. His half-baked ideas were leavened by a generous sprinkling of trust accorded his rank, without which, Brooks's malingering would have fallen flat.

Captain Brooks was emboldened by his early success at fooling people. His word as an officer, claiming illness, was accepted without question. Throwing caution to the wind, he recklessly increased the frequency and duration of his feigned illnesses. Murmurs of discontent began to percolate through the regiment but they never reached the ears of Captain Brooks, and his daring behavior continued unabated.

"Prior to his unit moving to the field he [Captain Brooks] reported to his commander that he 'was very sick and unable to proceed with his Regiment,' . . . he immediately thereafter entered upon a course of riotous living, attending balls, parties, picnics, dinner parties, etc."[40]

The dazzling social spotlight blinded Captain Brooks, and he remained unaware of the storm clouds building in the distance. His social omnipresence generated gossip and rumor concerning his liberal leave policy. Inevitably, his feigned illnesses boomeranged. Captain Brooks eventually met his fate in Boston, where he was apparently enjoying city life when a fellow acquaintance, surprised by the officer's presence, questioned him. Captain Brooks matter-of-factly responded that "he had been wounded in a battle in which his Regiment had recently been engaged, and that the wound was of such a nature, that he was obliged to use a cane." Brooks sought to convince his friend that the leave was convalescent in nature, but was unsuccessful, and military authorities arrested him.

A court-martial was convened charging Captain Brooks with the unauthorized absence and conduct unbecoming an officer and a gentleman. Witnesses who previously bore quiet reservations now vocally accused Brooks. Doubts about his many illnesses coalesced into certainty that they had been feigned. Oblivious, bold, or simply a rascal, Captain Brooks stoutly refuted his guilt.

Court-martial members listened intently to the prosecutor's case. Brooks had violated a sacred trust by dishonoring the officer corps. His behavior, according to the prosecutor, blemished all officers. When the parade of witnesses retired, the court-martial members deliberated Captain Brooks's fate and found him guilty as charged. His punishment was simple: "to be dismissed [from] the service of the U.S., and to be utterly disabled to have or to hold thereafter any office or employment in the service of the U.S."[41]

The relationship between cowardice and malingering was sometimes obvious. Many soldiers considered goldbricking just a notch above overt cowardice. The connection was clear when soldiers alternately resorted to both behaviors. The overlap between malingering and cowardice worked to the extreme disadvantage of soldiers suffering legitimate, but vague, disabilities.

Capt. Richard Lee was a volunteer member of the 8th Virginia Infantry Regiment. As a company commander, certain expectations were demanded of him. Honor, integrity, and bravery were essential ingredients of effective leadership, but Captain Lee squandered these attributes in a campaign of selfish shirking. The first inkling of concern about Captain Lee developed during an active military engagement. Captain Lee was observed to "leave his Company and go to the rear in a cowardly manner, his Company at the time being engaged with the enemy, and [he] did not rejoin his Company until after the action ceased."

Perhaps fellow soldiers initially discounted this shameless display, the general reservoir of faith in officers serving to quench any doubts. Lee might have offered a semiplausible explanation, perhaps citing some battlefield condition warranting his attention. In all probability, gossip started chipping away at the commander's stonewalling, and Lee might have heard the sullen innuendoes. In any event, he chose a different path. Instead of succumbing to panic and risking another display of cowardice, Lee charted a course of deception.

Captain Lee resorted to a simple ruse. While, "in command of the Regiment . . . [Captain Lee] chew[ed] tobacco, and used other means to make himself sick in a cowardly manner, that he might have an excuse for avoiding the coming engagement with the enemy." Captain Lee's deception was quickly identified, as he was already under suspicion from his prior act. The military acted swiftly, and Lee was charged with six specifications of cowardice, to which he plead not guilty. A brief trial ended Captain Lee's lackluster career. He was convicted and dismissed from service.[42]

There were different shades of malingering. Some of the darkest examples were prosecuted, but these were few in number. The decision to prosecute any crime was based on certain calculations, and, usually, the nature of the offense was pivotal. The weasel-like malingerer was despicable, but desertion was a more important military crime to prosecute. There were other factors to consider as well. The cost of a trial was measured in terms of the number of personnel who had to be diverted from other duties. It was simply too inconvenient to prosecute all types of misconduct. Malingering facilitated an untold number of deserters, and most were never captured. The unfortunate ones faced desertion charges—not malingering charges. Occasionally, malingering alone was too egregious to ignore.

Pvt. James Griffin, Company E, 5th Infantry, was charged with "malingering conduct, prejudicial to good order and military discipline." The allegations followed a most determined career. In a short space he "reported on sick-call 7 times with in the last 3 months, neither time of which, he, Private J. Griffin, is believed to have been sick."

Private Griffin employed a variety of ruses, none too clever. In one instance, he "complain[ed] that he had sprained his ankle while on fatigue duty, and that he was suffering from the same unable to walk, this being a false statement . . . not having suffered any injury on his ankle."

Soldiers were expected to get along with each other. When passions boiled over and fists started flying, both parties ultimately risked military punishment. Injuries from these physical imbroglios were used as evidence of misconduct. Surgeons heard many fanciful stories accounting for these bruises, bumps, and scratches. Private Griffin seized the opportunity to exploit an injury from a fight. The soldier shamelessly "report[ed] at sick-call with a deformed finger, stating that he had just broken or disjointed the same working with the ice . . . and did thereby obtain an excuse from duty, the same finger having been partially broken in a fight with another soldier."

Private Griffin sorely aggravated the surgeon, who wasted no time communicating his displeasure to the regimental commander, who, in turn, promptly arrested Griffin and put him under guard. In an effort to blunt the danger he faced, Private Griffin quickly admitted to one episode of malingering. It was a useless gesture; he was convicted of seven specifications of malingering when other instances came to light. The court-martial ordered Griffin "confined at hard labor for 3 months and . . . [to] forfeit $10 of his monthly pay for the same period."[43]

The military provided many motivations for malingering: hazardous duty, separation from family, limited furloughs, poor food, and unwholesome recreation. Every person who donned the uniform, to varying degrees, understood the environment—and what could grow in it. Most soldiers were resilient and succeeded despite the conditions; however, a substantial minority did not, forcing the military to confront vague boundaries between madness, malingering, and malfeasance. Eventually this exercise helped sharpen the lines between emotional and malevolent behavior.

CHAPTER SIX

────◆────

TRIALS OF MADNESS

Most cases presented to a court-martial resulted in conviction. The few remaining examples included acquittals or the rarely successful insanity defense. Among the small group of mentally disturbed offenders, there were two common dispositions. When evidence of mental instability was obvious, criminal charges might be dropped, and the prisoner could be released from military service, or if severely ill, transferred to a hospital. In a few cases the insanity defense was fully litigated.

In one brief illustration, Pvt. Thomas Seymore, Company C, 1st Michigan Colored Volunteers, was on guard duty when wanderlust struck him. He was subsequently charged with desertion. His obligatory appearance before a court-martial was embarrassing. It was painfully clear to the jury members that Private Seymore was mentally impaired: He presented with gross intellectual impairment, a speech impediment, and a childlike demeanor. At the conclusion of the brief trial, jury members considered the situation. Seymore had committed a crime, but the military shared some responsibility. He was not medically fit for duty, and a more discriminating recruitment physical should have determined that. The verdict seemed to recognize military

duplicity. The court found the accused, "Guilty, but attach no criminality there to . . . because the soldier is utterly deficient in mental
capacity. . . . The evidence showing the prisoner to be an idiot, he
will be released from imprisonment, and steps taken for his discharge
from the service."[1]

Andrew Overstreet was a private in Company C of the 38th U.S.
Infantry. Like Private Seymore, Overstreet was charged with quitting
his guard duty. He was also accused of selling military property, spe-
cifically a musket and forty rounds of ammunition. During the
arraignment when "called upon to plead, his conduct, and replies to
the questions asked him, were of such a character as to indicate that
he was at the time insane." Whether from suspiciousness or thoroughness the court launched an investigation, and witnesses who
knew Overstreet were called to testify. Some had a several-year history of association to relate. There was a compelling consistency in
the witnesses' description of Overstreet's behavior.

Private Overstreet suffered from episodic insanity, according to
some witnesses, dating back to his childhood. Verifying a link to earlier mental problems reinforced the validity of Private Overstreet's
current condition, and the court-martial members were satisfied that
his misconduct occurred during a recurring fit of insanity. At the time
of the trial, he was still insane, and to continue legal proceedings
would be pointless. The indictment was abandoned, and the trial
dismissed.[2]

The case of Pvt. Jeremiah Nolan created a different legal
dilemma. He was charged with a violation of the Forty-second Article
of War: "Any officer or soldier who misbehaves himself before the
enemy, runs away, or shamefully abandons any fort, post, or guard,
which he is commanded to defend, or speaks words inducing others
to do the like, or casts away his arms or ammunition, or quits his post
or colors to plunder or pillage, shall suffer death, or such other punishment as a court-martial may direct."[3]

Military legal procedure adhered to specific rules, one of which
required a plea be formally recorded during arraignment. If the
accused could not, or would not, enter a plea, the specter of a men-

tally incompetent soldier might haunt the fairness of the trial. This conundrum had frustrated English courts for years.[4] Various ways to overcome a nonpleading defendant, ranging from torture, to entering a guilty plea when the defendant refused to plead, to having the accused medically examined, were employed in the common law courts. American military courts responded to this rare event by directing a not guilty plea for the uncooperative prisoner. Occasionally, a physician would testify.

Private Nolan responded to the court-martial entreaties with stubbornness. His reluctance to plead was obstinately based on one point: He had never been read the Articles of War. Frustrated, the court again demanded Private Nolan either plead guilty or not guilty, but Private Nolan was not moved. "Still answering foreign to the purpose, the court directed the plea of not guilty to be recorded." The court having cleared this hurdle, the trial began in earnest.

The usual brevity characterized Private Nolan's trial. A more sophisticated inquiry might have explored the reason for Nolan's refusal to plea. On the surface it seemed obvious: The accused was attempting a clever defense strategy based on ignorance of the law. This was not a pointless ruse, since military authorities were required to provide a periodic public notice about the Articles of War. Private Nolan's objection received short shrift. Whether his stubborn refusal to submit to the court-martial had any basis in mental deficiency was similarly ignored. There was no medical testimony given in the trial.

Private Nolan was convicted—clearly the verdict reflected the jury members' opinion that willfulness, and not madness, governed Nolan. As a result he was "confined at hard labor . . . wearing a 12 lb. ball attached to his left leg, by a chain 3' long, for 3 months; and to forfeit $6/month of his pay, for the same period."[5]

Mental competency was a legal principle central to the conduct of a court-martial. A fair trial required that the accused understand the charges and have the mental facility to mount a defense. Insanity or idiocy robbed the prisoner of that capacity. During arraignment, the accused soldier was formally charged with criminal misconduct. At this time the defendant had the opportunity to assert innocence or seek mercy if guilty. If no plea was offered, the court was stuck, because strict legal rules prevented the trial from proceeding.[6] A pause was declared, and the recess continued until the court determined which of two reasons explained the failure to plead: Was the accused mute "from visitation from God" (the court's term for insanity) or mute from malice? If the court was convinced that madness prevented the defendant's participation in the trial, either medical treatment or discharge from military duty followed. Soldiers mute from malice suffered a different fate. Their actions were deemed willful, the court-martial would circumvent their obstinacy by imposing a not guilty plea, and the trial would resume. The case of Pvt. Joseph Hamley graphically depicted this process—and the consequence of disturbing routine military practice.[7]

Private Hamley was undoubtedly confused, and, as he stood before the court-martial members, a vague dread probably enveloped him. Something bad was happening. When an officer stood up and accused Hamley of military misconduct, his anxiety-driven confusion only worsened. After a brief pause, the soldier was repeatedly asked, "Private Hamley, how do you plea?" In Hamley's infantile mind, he probably assumed that since all these people were angry with him, he must have done something wrong. In response to the badgering Hamley finally mumbled "guilty."

The trial of Private Hamley was shameful. Witnesses were assembled, and they dutifully testified, one after another agreeing that Private Hamley lived "in a state of idiocy." Some openly wondered about his fitness for military duty, while others obliquely criticized his enlistment. Remarkably, the military court ignored the evidence of mental deficiency. Perhaps zeal to punish or a lack of familiarity with military law explained the rush to judgment. If the court members had any reservations about proceeding, they were not chronicled in the official transcripts. The jury demanded retribution despite what must have been an obviously mentally disturbed prisoner. Fortunately, this miscarriage of justice was corrected.

Military law granted an important safeguard, in the form of an automatic review of court-martial decisions. In this instance, the trial of Private Hamley drew an unusually stern rebuke. "If the Court had knowledge of this fact, it should have been considered before the arraignment, and the case dismissed. Persons of unsound mind are not supposed to be responsible for their acts, and are not legally subject to trial and punishment. The accused will be released from arrest."[8]

A cavalier approach was all too common in many courts-martial, and, regrettably, the very foundation of military justice was threatened by this unchecked attitude. The number of trials, mostly for desertion, seemed to invite shortcuts, because assembling officers, procuring evidence, and deliberating punishment were collectively time consuming. In the pressure to fight a war, expedience took priority over honoring strict legal rules, but, unfortunately, subverting established traditions increased the risk of an unjust outcome. The courts-martial system might have collapsed had not prudent action shored up the weakened structure. Halfway through the Civil War, Maj. Gen. George G. Meade, the Commanding General of the Army of the Potomac, intervened. In a sternly worded statement, the Commanding General complained, "After the proceedings have been confirmed and execution ordered, testimony has been brought forward which should have been developed before the Court. . . . It is not understood how Courts and Judge Advocates acting under the solemnity of an oath, and with the life of a fellow soldier depending on their action, can be so criminally negligent."[9]

The General was not satisfied with merely rebuking the legal system. Adherence to amazingly simple practices was demanded. Their absence hinted at the decay the court-martial process had succumbed to. "In cases of alleged desertion . . . it ought, if possible, to be shown when, where, and under what circumstances the apprehension took place; whether the accused was in uniform or citizens clothes . . . the story he told when arrested; in short, everything tending to show the intention of the accused."[10]

Concern was also emerging that mentally disordered soldiers were not receiving appropriate consideration. For political reasons alone, the military justice system could not stand to lose its credibility.

The sons of the Union Army came from families. If their voices of discontent were loud enough it could undermine popular support for the war. In a final order to his army, the Commanding General of the Army of the Potomac demanded that, "If there is any reason to suppose he is deficient in intellect, the testimony of Medical Officers should be taken as to his mental condition."[11]

This final, and liberal injunction was probably doomed to a minor role. Forces pushing for speedy trials would see medical testimony as a time-consuming hindrance. Furthermore, medical officers were extremely busy and not particularly agreeable to performing an additional duty.

The Commanding General's bluntness was unusual. Very few authorities considered linking mental impairment with criminal behavior. When juries deliberated a capital case, the stakes were even higher. Once again, the general expressed his concern. "The accused should be made fully to understand the critical situation in which he is placed, and every facility should be given him to introduce testimony in his defense."[12] Regrettably, some trials did just the opposite.

Pvt. Simon Kennedy killed Pvt. James Fitzgerald. Kennedy's story was dryly summarized in a brief general order issued by the Department of the Pacific in 1864. "Private Simon Kennedy of Company 'D,' Third Artillery did assault with a deadly weapon, intending to kill" Pvt. James Fitzgerald. Another soldier, Pvt. Michael Condon suffered grievous wounds at the hand of Kennedy but survived. The facts in this case were essentially uncontested, in spite of the irrationality of the crime combined with notable legal errors committed by the court-martial. Kennedy was charged with murder even though the alleged facts did not support the legal definition. The man killed, Private Fitzgerald, was a close friend of his attacker. Both victims, Fitzgerald and Condon, were assaulted "in the night time after all had laid down to sleep." In addition, an embarrassing admission about Kennedy "shows culpable carelessness on the part of the guard in suffering arms to be in the possession of men in confinement, and particularly when a man [Kennedy] was . . . suffering from mental derangement." Unhindered by any objections, the trial proceeded without much delay. No one heeded the Commanding General's sage advice "to introduce testimony" beneficial to the defense.[13]

Private Kennedy was convicted of murder, but the court exercised a measure of compassion and imposed a life sentence. Perhaps the sentence reflected the jury's fainthearted stab at justice; if so it was a useless gesture. The court-martial collapsed on appeal. In a fitting turn of events, the trial was condemned and the prisoner properly released. The reviewing officer sounded an incredulous tone. "The charge of murder is not sustained . . . there being no malice aforethought or premeditation or indeed intent, of any kind alleged. The evidence shows that the killing of Fitzgerald, and the stabbing of Condon, were neither preceded nor accompanied by any altercation, quarrel, or even abusive language; the man killed was a friend."[14] The lack of criminal intent was puzzling. To satisfy his curiosity, the reviewing officer dug deeper. The answer lay on the surface of the detailed trial record. Private Kennedy was mentally unsound and there was "abundant evidence to show the acts were committed whilst the prisoner was insane."[15] The trial court failed Kennedy by not introducing any evidence regarding his mental state. Fortunately the failsafe mechanism of review corrected the error. The sentence was dismissed and in its place, the reviewing officer ordered Private Kennedy "be held in confinement till he can be sent to the insane asylum."[16]

There were countless courts-martial that were conducted without following even rudimentary legal procedure. This haste to convict left little time for serious preparation. Only the most blatant miscarriages of justice earned a rebuke. In part, that was attributable to the nascent interest in mental disorders. Mental illness was a new concept making inroads into medical thinking. The Civil War magnified the significance of emotional health. Military recruitment and retention were both negatively impacted by novel, often inexplicable, ailments, many of which, over time, were accepted as mental disorders. Three diagnoses were eventually included among that small group: nostalgia, psychosomatic illness, and insanity. The slow growth of knowledge about these diseases had partially resulted from stagnation in

general medical education and poor military health care. Both, paradoxically, were invigorated by the demands of a nation at war.

Military medicine was a lethal weapon during the early years, with
untold numbers of soldiers needlessly suffering and even perishing.
In some cases the reckless acts of military surgeons took a toll.[17] The
culprit was a poorly organized health care delivery system.[18] Lack of
ambulances left evacuation to the mercy and caprice of fellow troops.
When operational necessity forced a retreat or the numbers of
wounded overwhelmed relief efforts, the unfortunate victims suffered
where they fell, and many died a slow, agonizing death.

The military struggled mightily, usually in vain, to improve medical care. Public pressure was needed. The process started informally,
with tales of suffering attracting visitors and volunteer nurses to the
general hospitals. Energized by compassion, the volunteers in particular demanded better conditions. Individual voices soon coalesced and
influential agencies were born; among these, the Sanitary Commission was preeminent.[19]

Women volunteered their labor in many northern cities and provided clothing, food, and nursing care. Doctors joined the crusade
and, in one instance, founded the Medical Association for Furnishing
Hospital Supplies. These well-intentioned medical support efforts
were hampered through a lack of organization. Each local group
influenced only a small portion of the total war effort. Maximum
impact required a national vision.

A group of prominent citizens, many from New York, were determined to build a national relief agency, which they named the Sanitary Commission. Many hours and late nights culminated in a list of
recommendations of ways to improve the efficiency of medical care.
The Sanitary Commission placed prevention at the top of their list:
Illness could be reduced with proper military attention to diet, camp
hygiene, recreational pursuits, and medical care.

The original members of the Sanitary Commission were men
accustomed to wielding power. Their influence opened doors, and
they sought to press their cause to the highest levels of government.
President Lincoln was receptive and invited them to the White

House. The President listened sympathetically, as the members of the Sanitary Commission outlined their vision. It was a powerful message, and Lincoln granted his enthusiastic stamp of approval.

The Sanitary Commission was chartered to examine recruiting practices, field hygiene, and the health care system. The Commission's authority was limited to a strictly advisory role. Perhaps a weaker group would have faltered without more control, but the members of the Sanitary Commission were fearless. They successfully lobbied Congress for changes. If the military hoped to hobble the high-minded outsiders, they seriously underestimated the Commission's fervor.

The sorry state of the military medical organization was an early target of the Sanitary Commission. Competent medical officers were put in command, and plans were developed to build modern military hospitals. The ranks of the Sanitary Commission swelled with each victory. To monitor progress, the Sanitary Commission used inspectors, who served as the eyes and ears of the organization. Their reports contributed to a predictable infusion of medical supplies, ambulances, and nurses.

The Sanitary Commission could point with pride to yet another virtue: All expenses were funded through private donations. Charity drives were conducted with military precision, and vast sums poured into Sanitary Commission coffers. Sanitary Commission fairs were creative and profitable fund-raisers, which typically drew enthusiastic crowds. Fair goers were treated to livestock shows, auctions, country cooking, and dealers hawking all manner of goods.

As a result military medical care improved. The relentless pressure of the Sanitary Commission, joined by similar minded groups, left little wiggle room. Congress and military leaders bowed to the wishes of these powerful interests. These compassionate citizens understood a simple reality—illness felled more soldiers than bullets. As a result, their energies were predominately directed toward reducing physical illness and injuries. However, their success was partially countered by a troubling development—the emotional cost of the war. The long neglected debt piled up, and the military paid dearly for this oversight.

Patriotic fervor underwrote the initial massive enlistment. Soldiers on both sides expected a short conflict, but, as the war relentlessly dragged on, a number of realities intruded. Chief among these were the consequences of combat: death and maiming. Adding to the risk of violent death was the utter absence of many creature comforts that were taken for granted in civilian life. Field conditions were primitive. Conditions of crowding, compounded by poor hygiene and poor camp sanitation, resulted in the easy spread of disease. Typhoid, dysentery, and lesser ills raced through the ranks. Those soldiers that succumbed to illness had a bleak future. Hope of recovery was often dashed by the reality of limited medical care. The numbers of suffering victims confirmed rumors of poor medical support.

The misery and boredom of military life was poorly pacified. Recreational pursuits were limited and harmful. Alcohol, gambling, and prostitutes were readily available diversions, but pleasure came at the expense of rampant venereal disease and the danger of punishment for misconduct.

The best military commanders understood that effective leadership hinged on balancing the deprivations of war with esprit de corps. A proper blend produced an elusive motivational force that ensured an unswerving loyalty. Such devotion inured soldiers, cloaking them with an umbrella-like protection, and resulted in a decline in the number of injuries, illness, and incidents of misconduct. Conversely, military units plagued with poor leadership, low morale, and indiscipline experienced substantially higher rates of attrition. Students of military science were quick to grasp a key concept: Healthy commands produced healthy troops—better immunized against illness, injury, pessimism, and above all, emotional casualties.

Recognizing the emotional casualties of war was difficult, and enormously complicated when mental anguish masqueraded as physical illness or misconduct. Overt expression of fear, anxiety, or depression was not tolerated and was answered by ridicule and debasement more often than sympathy. A major factor preventing widespread acceptance of emotional problems was their ease of fabrication. Vague physical symptoms were sometimes greeted with suspicion, and soldiers with a history of goldbricking were obvious targets of derision.

The fainthearted resorted to various displays of emotion: battlefield paralysis, confusion, sobbing, whimpering, whining, or simply hiding, and they were branded as cowards. When terror led to flight, the charge was desertion. Military law functioned as a rod adding rigidity to a timorous soldier's backbone. Two moral forces, punishment and social disgrace, acted in tandem to overcome a weak will, but it was not a uniformly effective military practice. In some cases, bottled passions were uncorked through intemperance. Emotional distress underwent a psychosomatic transformation in other soldiers. The most dramatic expression was a raw display of psychotic despair.

A host of factors played on the soldier's spirit. Confidence, in fellow soldiers and commanders, was crucial. For many, the unnecessary delay in pay was a chronic irritant. Poor victuals guaranteed grousing. The miseries of boredom, bad weather, filth, illness, and injury were exceeded by only one deprivation—silence from home.

The deprivations of war demanded emotional adaptation, and a common cathartic was letter writing. Letters from home were always eagerly anticipated, because, through them, for a few moments, the reader could be transported from the battlefield to home. Tender thoughts expressed on paper mitigated the physical separation. Real hardships were softened, and no tonic could soothe an embattled soul better. The soldier and his family were both strengthened by the words.

Cruel, insensitive communication could cut deeper than any weapon. Wounds were inflicted through heart-wrenching silence, plaintive pleas that selfishly ignored the plight of the reader, Dear John letters, or imperious demands. Mail call could surprise the unsuspecting reader with an emotional landmine. One soldier lamented, "Before we was married I heard from you every week and now we married I don't hear from you once a month."[20]

The irregular process of granting furloughs coupled longing with bitterness. It also magnified the importance of letter writing, particularly in those soldiers more vulnerable to emotional decompensation. Some commanders routinely denied applications for leave, which was a shortsighted approach. In such instances, it was inevitable that the soldiers would make comparisons between home life and camp deprivation, which, in turn, forced many soldiers to think about desertion. Commanders understood the risk and responded with a predictable tightening of military control. A somber mood smothered these units, and the first casualty was the commander's most important commodity—respect of his troops. Training, discipline, and combat performance steadily withered in such a noxious environment.

Smart officers realized that leadership and victory were crafted from a balance of emotional and military motivations. As Gen. Joseph Shields confided, "if not allowed to go home and see their families . . . [soldiers] . . . droop and die."[21]

Pvt. Ezra Bingham, Company G, 161st Ohio, was never a happy soul. The normal passions of life, such as ecstasy and love, had bypassed him. Military service only deepened his despair. His sleep grew increasingly tortured, and terrible nightmares caused him to toss about endlessly each night. Private Bingham sank into emotional quicksand.[22] The change in Bingham was gradual, but eventually his friends grew concerned. He began to avoid typical diversions, such as cards and music, which he had previously enjoyed. Private Bingham was emotionally bankrupt; it was as if all pleasure had been struck from his life.

Bingham lost the most obvious mark of a soldier next—the art of complaining. Hard work and boredom generally worked together to sharpen a soldier's appetite, and grumbling was the universal condiment that seasoned the usually unpalatable fare. Private Bingham was in a listless, dazed state, and he neither groused about nor ate his food. Bingham lost weight as his appetite plummeted, he developed a hacking cough, and eventually disease overwhelmed his weakened defenses.

Private Bingham was unable to muster the strength to arise one morning, claiming his entire body ached. A sympathetic sergeant alerted the surgeon, and Private Bingham was evacuated to a hospital. On admission he was "much depressed in spirits and exceedingly homesick."[23]

A few months passed with no improvement. The hospital record dispassionately recorded the disquieting turn in Bingham's condition. "His pulse was weak, cough slight, expectoration tough and stringy, skin dry and harsh, tongue white; hectic fever, dysphagia and much prostration were followed by hiccough, and death."[24] Private Bingham died from depression.

Many military surgeons carefully reported their medical findings. Successful surgical procedures were trumpeted in journals and by word of mouth. Diseases were catalogued. The more astute doctors sought explanations and treatments for the novel conditions confronting them. Obviously, no remedy that depleted military manpower was seriously suggested. Prevention and treatment had to be reconciled with recruiting, retention, deployments, limited furloughs, and even erratic mail delivery.

Not all surgeons abided by these informal rules. One heretical physician criticized the "evils of youthful enlistments."[25] Dr. DeWitt Peters, an assistant surgeon, bravely bucked prevailing wisdom and focused on youthful recruits. He carefully set forth several reasons decrying young enlistments. Dr. Peters was convinced that eighteen-year-old soldiers lacked the stamina required for military duty. He fervently believed that, confronted with the deprivations of military service, these youngsters quickly succumbed through illness. The problem was worsened by the perfunctory induction physicals, which recruits easily passed, even when serious medical conditions existed.

The naïveté of young recruits generally ensured a successful appeal to their patriotism. In addition, there was a scarcely concealed campaign to romanticize military service. Visions of glory tempted many, but once they were ensnared, the reality of army life dispelled the fantasies. Although most soldiers persevered in spite of the disillusionment, a respectable minority could not adapt. "In a few months the novelty of long marches, guard duty, exposure, and innumerable hardships, has vanished, [the soldier's] mind begins to despond, and the youth is now a fair victim for fever or some other terrible scourge that is to wreck his constitution and blight his hopes."[26] The syndrome was fairly common and certainly unique to military service. It was most often associated with homesickness, justifying the medical label of nostalgia.

Nostalgia was recognized in the military medical literature as a peculiar condition of the mind.[27] It seemed to represent a new category of mental illness. Insanity and melancholia were two widely acknowledged mental disorders. Nostalgia was conceptualized on a continuum, ranging from severe depression of the spirits to insanity. It was the clearly induced nature of the malady that puzzled physicians. The condition invariably developed after the susceptible soldier left home. The unrelenting, downhill spiral of nostalgia fostered comparisons with insanity. Curiously though, a complete reversal in symptoms followed the soldier's return home. Traditional medical beliefs were challenged; insanity and melancholy rarely responded in such a predictable manner. Nostalgia had many facets, with doctors variously seeing depression, madness, or malingering. The diagnosis depended on the opinion of the individual surgeon.

Soldiers afflicted with nostalgia would weep inconsolably, obstinately refuse proffered tinctures and tonics, and then decline precipitously in physical health. An astute surgeon wrote, "Fresh troops serving in the extreme South, where mail communications are irregular, and where the climate is very debilitating suffer terribly this affliction. . . . The majority of them were young men from the Eastern states, whose love of home and kindred is a characteristic trait."[28]

A sense of urgency forced the military medical system to respond. The absolute number of reported cases remained small, yet an almost irrational fear seized some military planners: Nostalgia seemed infectious.

Early efforts aimed at treating nostalgia were experimental in nature. Surgeons naturally focused their energies on the physical presentation of the syndrome. Creative tonics were formulated but none were universally accepted—or successful—and hope for a simple pharmacological cure dwindled. Nostalgia only responded to a more comprehensive treatment program. After gaining several years experience with the disorder, some surgeons promoted a workable treatment plan.

The disabling version of homesickness labeled nostalgia curiously spared some units. This patchwork distribution was carefully scrutinized, and it was determined that military outfits distinguished by high morale, firm discipline, and fair leadership suffered fewer cases of nostalgia. Occupation of the mind was the tonic that relieved morbid preoccupations. Rigorous military training acted like a trusted sentry guarding the mind. Debilitating thoughts were repelled, never gaining a conscious foothold. Techniques designed for prevention were adapted for treatment. The remedies were borne from paradoxical observations. "Kind and sympathizing words—amusements— seemed to invite a more deplorable condition. . . . No ordinary means could arouse them from their mental and physical inactivity."[29] Surgeons eventually made the connection. Factors that promoted nostalgia, such as inactivity, could be countered by a thoughtful plan. "The patients are now required to exercise to the extent of their physical ability. This was enjoined as a duty. At the same time, a system was inaugurated to impress them that their disease was a moral turpitude; that soldiers of courage, patriotism and sense should be superior to the influences that brought about their condition."[30]

Under this new regimen, nostalgia was managed with a mixture of cajoling, shame, and forced labor. No longer was sympathy de rigueur. The normal rules of etiquette allowed sick people to receive special favors, but benefits such as reduced work obligations, better food, or simply a secure resting spot, were denied patients with nostalgia. This change in tactics upset many victims, and they responded angrily.

One medical author, urging the tough approach to nostalgia, trumpeted his results. "Within two years not a single case of Nostalgia has occurred . . . the odium attached to the disease has played a part in causing men to overcome the influence which tend to its production."[31]

The powerful motivations underlying homesickness might be

temporarily channeled but not eliminated. Soldiers feigning nostalgia might drop the ruse as the social cost increased; however, the more seriously afflicted did not respond to bullying tactics. As one medical author accurately noted, "In cases where complications exist, notwithstanding [the surgeon's] zealous efforts, the symptoms will frequently baffle his skill, and then . . . in order to save life . . . he must recommend the man's discharge.[32]

Nostalgia was a medical conundrum that only a few physicians sought to unravel. The condition lay somewhere between real illness and malingering, an area occupied by an emerging field of study called psychosomatics. A few enlightened physicians undertook the study of psychosomatic medicine, but most doctors derisively dismissed the nervous soldier as involved in nothing more than a willful charade. Bucking this trend were physicians like Dr. S. Weir Mitchell, who was convinced that nerve injuries and nervous disorders were real and treatable. Army Surgeon General William A. Hammond was infected by their enthusiasm. This enlightened medical leader demonstrated his support by authorizing a hospital solely dedicated to the study and treatment of nerve injuries. Turner's Lane Hospital in Philadelphia soon enjoyed a full quota of four hundred patients.[33]

The reputation of Turner's Lane Hospital spread rapidly. The enthusiasm of Dr. Mitchell and his associates was like a magnet drawing patients from exasperated military surgeons. The average military surgeon had very little patience for nervous ailments. The usual nostrums did little, and disgruntled, disaffected patients remained as reminders of their failure. If nothing else, Turner's Lane served to remove these baffling patients from embarrassed military surgeons.

Mitchell and his associates prospered from these outcasts, while optimism and creative treatments greeted the desperate sufferers. For many patients, Turner's Lane Hospital promised hope. "As the wounded of each period of the war have been cured, discharged, invalided, or died, every large hospital has had left among the wards two or three or more strange instances of wounds of nerves. Most of them presented phenomena which are rarely seen, and which were naturally foreign to the observation even of those surgeons whose experience was the most extensive and complete."[34]

Among the hospital dregs sent to Turner's Lane were nerve injuries that initially defied even Dr. Mitchell's comprehension. These dead-end evaluations always yielded the same outcome. Despite the appearance of disabling physical symptoms, the diagnostic examination was entirely normal. All organ systems were functioning properly. Mitchell and his colleagues pushed the boundaries of convention with such riddles. Inevitably, these intrepid explorers entered the uncharted terrain of human behavior. No scalpel could dissect the layers of human behavior. This intellectual obstacle created an impediment the average physician could not surmount; however, Dr. Mitchell and company responded to this challenge by adopting a holistic approach.

The majority of Civil War Era physicians believed in dualism, which held that the mind and body were separate entities. Physical ailments, like their mental counterparts, developed independent of each other. The concepts of mind and soul were interchangeable. This left the treatment of erratic behavior to a decidedly nonmedical group. Family, friends, chaplains, and a host of charlatans filled the space left by medical neglect. Physicians focused almost exclusively on physical aliments, rarely connecting mental illness with organic dysfunction. Dr. Mitchell rejected the popular mind-body dualism. Instead, he proposed an integrated mind-body paradigm, which explained how emotions and physical symptoms were inseparably intertwined. It was an important advance.

Dr. Mitchell's theory of a mind-body unity removed an obstacle to understanding mental disorders. Physicians could no longer ignore the emotional side of their patients. "The mental attitudes of the nervous man demand of his physician the most careful attention, nor can we afford to disregard anything in his ways of life or his habits of thought and action. We must determine for him how far and how much he shall use his mind; whatever it be, what his amusements should be. The careful student of such cases will find in the individuality of his cases the need for the most minute of such studies, and, above all, he will learn that, the more fully he commands the confidence of his patient the more can he effect. Such people are greatly helped by a word or two of decisive promise or reassurance."[35]

Dr. Mitchell's progressive thinking was hobbled by his tendency to blur moral turpitude with mental disorders. This attitude imperceptibly colored his treatment philosophy. Mitchell considered drugs a last resort for nervous conditions. Medications had a role in alleviating physical discomfort, but moral defects required a different approach. Procedures that Mitchell found effective for nerve injuries were adapted for "confirmed cases of hysteria."

Hysteria was a relatively ambiguous term, which was loosely defined as a physical disorder without an apparent organic etiology. Hysteria was not clearly distinguished from psychosomatic disorders, and just about every known physical disease had a psychosomatic counterpart.

Dr. Mitchell used mild electrical stimulation to foster nerve regeneration, and he achieved remarkable results in restoring long lost muscle activity. Both patients and practitioners cheered the outcome. Given the gray area between real disease and psychosomatic illness, it seemed logical to apply the proven technique to both conditions. Results were less impressive with the psychosomatic patients.

Dr. Mitchell's real innovation was his "rest cure." Patients suffering a psychosomatic illness were treated to a vigorous "effort to lift the health of patients to a higher plane by the use of seclusion, which cuts off excitement and foolish sympathy; by rest . . . by massage . . . and by electrical muscular excitation."[36] Coupled with the rest cure were steadfast injunctions urging the sufferer to assume responsibility for the illness. Dr. Mitchell would advise the patient to "be strong" or assert their "masculinity."

Mitchell was not alone in exploring the frontiers of mental disease. The medical literature documented the efforts of other medical pioneers. Dr. J. M. Da Costa reported one common and curious disability. Writing in the *American Journal of the Medical Sciences*, Dr. Da Costa presented an article entitled "On Irritable Heart:

A Clinical Study of a Form of Functional Cardiac Disorder and Its Consequences."[37]

Da Costa, like Mitchell, specialized in managing obscure cases shunned by most physicians. Once again, infectious zeal was transmitted throughout the local military district, and a bounty of medical cases was sent to receive his care.

Dr. Da Costa described many of his two hundred cases in painstaking detail. A general syndrome emerged from the collection of referrals he received. The symptoms Da Costa recognized arose primarily in seasoned combatants. The psychosomatic disorder that Da Costa studied began rather innocuously. Diarrhea and fever were the initial complaints, both of which progressively worsened. Sufferers eventually received a medical evacuation from their unit, and a short stay in the hospital seemingly cured the problem. Soldiers begged to leave the hospital, and the surgeon gladly appeased their wishes to rejoin their units.

Innumerable examples of diarrhea and fever flooded military medical facilities, and an appalling number of soldiers either died or suffered lingering debility from it. Da Costa's group appeared sturdier, and they were generally eager to rejoin their former units. The twist came when they returned. Almost immediately after the soldiers resumed their former responsibilities, a creeping invalidism surfaced. Any physical activity, including marches and drills, led quickly to utter exhaustion. The least exertion induced palpitations, breathlessness, headaches, dizziness, and chest pain.

Casualties overwhelmed military surgeons, and most had little time or patience for puzzles. Dr. Da Costa was the beneficiary. The soldiers were removed from battle and safely nestled in a hospital, where they underwent intense physical diagnostic scrutiny focused on their hearts. All symptoms eventually faded except those of presumed cardiac origin. The victims were obsessed with a panicky preoccupation of imminent heart failure; otherwise, they experienced a full recovery from physical symptoms. Dr. Da Costa dubbed the crippling cardiac condition an "irritable heart."

Irritable heart implied a functional or nervous etiology. Dr.

Da Costa freely admitted, "Holding at the time the common belief that functional and organic affections are widely separate, I failed at first to seize the fact that the apparently dissimilar states were in reality one. . . . But as patients multiplied I began to trace the connection."[38]

Da Costa's curiosity was piqued, and he launched a full-scale clinical study. Over the next few months, Dr. Da Costa carefully recorded and reported his observations on two hundred cases. Demographic data were collected, sorted, and analyzed. Age, occupation, and habits were among a long list of questions asked of each soldier. From the data Da Costa hoped to mine a wealth of discoveries.

Pvt. William O., a member of the New York Volunteers, was a typical example of an irritable heart patient. The soldier was twenty-one years old, and before donning the uniform, he was employed as a farmer. Shortly after commencing military duty, Pvt. William O. was stricken with diarrhea, and he gamely bore the malady for months. On a large march across Virginia, palpitations and shortness of breath compounded his misery. Determined not to quit, Pvt. William O. was finally felled by a severe cold, and he lost his voice. The surgeon intervened at this point, and after a cursory evaluation, Private O. was evacuated to the care of Dr. Da Costa at Turner's Lane Hospital. Labeled as case 261, he became the subject of dispassionate study. "Appearance that of fair health; gums rather spongy, says that they bled easily while in the field . . . appetite good; bowels regular; respiration 24 in the minute; pulse 122; impulse of heart extended, and very jerky. . . . On lying down pulses become fuller, and is reduced to 98. . . . He is still aphonic."[39]

Dr. Da Costa reached deep into his materia medica. Gelsemium, oxide of zinc, and strychnia all failed to control the excitable heart. Digitalis calmed the anxious organ, but Da Costa placed little faith in it being a permanent cure. "It was evident that he would not be fit for active duty for a very long time, he was detailed as orderly."[40]

Nearly two-thirds of those diagnosed with an irritable heart were younger than twenty-five. Da Costa found no relationship between irritable heart and pre-military work. "Painter, butcher, blacksmith, carpenter, the city-bred man who had left his desk in the counting-house, the farmer fresh from tilling the fields, were all fully represented in the long list of sufferers."[41]

Dr. Da Costa searched carefully for connections that might explain the origin of irritable heart, and hard field service seemed to be the chief culprit. Long road marches and extended maneuvering with the enemy preceded most cases. The doctor was also convinced that masturbation and tobacco abuse dissipated the body defenses, making soldiers more susceptible. Fevers and diarrhea occurred in nearly half the cases. Rarely did an injury precipitate irritable heart, although there were notable exceptions, and Da Costa reported two such cases: a soldier struck by a sandbag over his heart and another "in a hand-to-hand encounter [was] hit on the left breast with the butt of a musket."[42]

The symptoms of irritable heart could not be neatly catalogued. Cardiac palpitations defined the disorder, but the other clinical symptoms varied somewhat. "In some the attacks lasted several hours. . . . They occurred at all times of the day and night. . . . Yet there were cases that did not have them for days at a time. The seizures were, of course, most readily excited by exertion. . . . But attacks also occurred when the patient was quietly in bed."[43] The majority of irritable heart sufferers had chest pain, headaches, and dizziness. Breathing was labored but not especially rapid, and involuntary movements and fretful dreams denied the victims restful sleep.

Dr. Da Costa experimented with several therapeutic interventions, and after numerous trials, the simplest most effective remedy was found to be rest. When patients were prescribed frequent periods of respite lasting several hours, the frequency of palpitations and associated complaints decreased.

The rest cure was supplemented by an assortment of drugs. Aconite and digitalis were found useful in settling the irritable heart. Belladonna, a potent anticholinergic, also slowed the heart, but it had constipation as a side effect. Tonics, with their high alcohol content, were naturally sedating, and a consequence of their use was the reduction of anxiety.

The symptoms of irritable heart did not yield to treatment quickly.

During the first few weeks of hospitalization, the heart continued its furious pounding. Dr. Da Costa's patients demanded intense, long-term care, but, eventually, the irritable heart symptoms subsided. This limited success paved the way for the soldier's return to duty, but Da Costa respected the fragile recovery, since a sudden immersion would scuttle the progress. He wisely lengthened the hospital treatment through an extended convalescence. Soldiers were returned to their former regiments with light duty orders.

A total of seventy-six soldiers successfully completed Da Costa's treatment, and they all returned to their respective regiments. A typical subject reported by Dr. Da Costa was "case 62." "Samuel" was a twenty-eight-year-old soldier who "never was able to do much marching, and had marked cardiac symptoms." Dr. Da Costa treated Samuel with rest, digitalis, and belladonna, and his symptoms improved sufficiently to justify a return to duty. "He joined his regiment, and marched with it for several months. . . . He had remained well, all [cardiac] irregularity had ceased."[44]

Da Costa discovered two important principles that shaped recovery from a nervous disorder: attitude and convalescence. Soldiers first admitted to the hospital fully expected their medical condition to justify a discharge from the Army. They soon realized otherwise—Dr. Da Costa anticipated recovery. Resistance to the inevitable return to duty was quelled with a firm subliminal message. Implicitly embedded in the treatment plan for each patient was the expectation of recovery and restoration of military fitness.

The ultimate mental derangement was insanity. Madness conjured up the most frightful visions. To make matters worse, it was poorly understood, unpredictable, and seemingly uncontrollable. The social reaction of the general public and medical treatment by doctors shared a decidedly ambiguous response. Historically, madness fell within the province of religion, and limited strides away from that thinking had been made. There still remained a hesitation assigning an unqualified medical status to insanity, in part tempered by a suspicion of the victim's complicity. Doubts about a medical etiology of madness conflicted with the lingering moral interpretation. In the religious view, a person's character acted as a shield deflecting corrupting influences. A good, strong moral fiber was the lifelong consequence of religious faith, and lax morals and sinful hedonism weakened the armor. A lifetime of overindulgence battered the soul. Collapse was inevitable, and madness was the punishment.

Against the dark, moral theory of insanity, a few bold physicians offered a different vision. This new pathway was illuminated by war. The light leading the way to a new discovery occurred when insanity followed a traumatic brain injury, and war provided numerous opportunities to study head injuries. Many cases involved penetrating skull wounds, whereas others were blast concussions. A surprising percentage developed significant emotional aftereffects. That observation fueled speculation that structural abnormalities of the brain were the basis for insanity.

The average surgeon was preoccupied with injuries and illness. Insanity was a rare distraction. Management, not research, was their interest. Another smaller group of academically inclined physicians placed a premium on the medical treatment of insanity. Both sides, for different reasons, clamored for public institutions to house the mentally ill. The lay citizenry joined the effort, welcoming the institution as a fortress protecting society from the unpredictable actions of madmen. Physicians were designated as directors of insane asylums, emphasizing the respect that was increasingly granted the scientific treatment of insanity.

However, nowhere was the schism between a moral or medical basis for insanity exploited more dramatically than in criminal trials. No middle ground was sought, as skilled advocates polarized the debate. Insanity trials were uncommon; even at the height of military mobilization, only a handful of military insanity cases were tried. In spite of their small numbers, insanity cases often sparked passionate debates. Prosecutors were generally unfamiliar with both the law and the mental disorder. Arguments might have been weak, but opposition was often nonexistent.

A shrewd prosecutorial strategy foisted a straw man line of reasoning. The prosecutor advanced the notion of madness—but only under the most stringent definition. According to the prosecutor, insanity applied only to the most depraved, beast-like behavior. The prosecution then systematically compared, and distinguished, the accused from that self-serving description. The goal was to reinterpret the defendant's criminal behavior as purposeful, not as irrational. Evidence of premeditation, planning, and escape were offered as proof of evil intent. Anger and vengeance were the usual motives the prosecution offered as an explanation for the criminal act.

A skilled defense attorney could easily counter the prosecution using two broad strategies: humanize the defendant and offer medical testimony. Convincing a skeptical jury that a defendant was not mentally responsible for his behavior was tricky. Success in part depended on the attorney demystifying mental illness. The attorney might argue that mental illness was a normal, but extreme, variation of human behavior. In this line of reasoning, even normal people, given sufficient pressure, could mentally buckle. Implicating a common vulnerability supposedly present in every person was a tactic used to link the defendant to the jury, and it was hoped this ploy stirred sympathetic feelings among the jury members. Empathic jury members might foresee insanity developing under certain conditions in everyone.

The other legal tactic was more direct. Defense attorneys offered medical testimony to counter the moral depravity argument. A physician might ascribe the defendant's behavior to mental delusions—specific false beliefs that usurped rational faculties. The victim was controlled by reality-distorting thoughts. Innocent gestures and idle gossip assumed menacing proportions when misinterpreted by the mentally deluded person. Under sway of this internal mental duress, the defense attorney insisted that the accused soldier lost all moral accountability for his behavior. He was sick and deserved treatment instead of punishment.

America had struggled since colonial times with mental illness.[45] Religious, moral, legal, and medical philosophies alternately assumed control. Early in American history, the mentally ill were often abandoned, left to aimlessly wander the country. When their behavior con-

flicted with society, jail became their home. Winds of reform from
Europe swept over America in the eighteenth century, replacing punishment with compassion as the force driving the care of the mentally
ill. A benign paternalism favored providing mentally ill patients with
care and a place to live. Hospitals were erected to house the insane,
and the raving, incoherent madman who was destitute, hungry, and
dangerous was provided a stable environment. The hospital environment promoted social behavior among inmates, and endless medical
experimentation sought a cure. Society pressed the battle against
mental illness, confident of victory. Optimism persuaded the U.S.
Congress to establish a national insane asylum.

The U.S. Congress approved the lofty sum of $100,000 in 1852
to purchase land for an insane asylum in our nation's capital. A few
years later, Congress provided the statutory language to organize the
asylum. The goal was to develop "the most humane care and enlightened curative treatment of the insane of the Army and Navy." The
U.S. Congress named the facility The Government Hospital for the
Insane. Beneficiaries included military members and the poor civilian
residents of Washington, D.C.[46]

Admissions to The Government Hospital for the Insane exploded
during the Civil War. Its prime location near the Virginia battlefields
offered a convenient evacuation facility. During the first full year of
the war, soldiers and sailors accounted for three-fourths of all admissions. Impatience, intolerance, and clinical inexperience accelerated
a trend favoring quick disposition of these behavioral misfits. Surgeons were relieved of a burden they scarcely understood.

The staff assigned to The Government Hospital for the Insane
took evident pride in their work, and physicians established the standard of care. In the prewar years, when patients were admitted to the
hospital, they were generally accompanied by a written description of
their mental condition. Local physicians, with the input of family and
friends, were able to construct a relatively complete story.

A legal petition often preceded admission to the Government
Hospital. Two physicians would certify the presence of a specific
mental disorder. Their signatures attested to a medical examination

supporting the need for involuntary hospitalization. The petition for hospitalization also required lay certification. Signatures by "house-holders and residents of the District of Columbia," acknowledged the patient's indigent status. A justice of the peace sanctioned the pro-ceeding. Satisfied that the twin conditions of destitution and insanity were proven, the justice would authorize the admission.[47]

The predictable procedures that brought civilian patients to the Government Hospital were disrupted by the Civil War. From the out-set of the war, military admissions progressively took the place of civilian referrals. One of the prime casualties from this displacement was communication. The exigencies of war and military medical inex-perience conspired to inhibit the flow of information. Soldiers received at the Government Hospital were accompanied by the flim-siest of written records, leaving the hospital vulnerable. It was futile to try to reconstruct the reason for admission by interviewing a patient with a delirious mind. The frustration bubbled over in an Annual Report of the Government Hospital: "Admissions during the year . . . almost uniformly disobey that article of the regulations which requires that a 'history of the cases' should be sent with insane sol-diers—and the person, commonly a soldier, detailed to accompany an insane comrade to the hospital, has usually been as unacquainted with the history of the mental disorder under which his charge labored as is a trooper with the past history of the horse that is allot-ted him."[48]

The Government Hospital for the Insane was an administrative division of the Department of Interior. Commanders seeking the admission of one of their soldiers to the Government Hospital could make direct appeals to the Interior Department. The request might be tersely drawn, with little more than the soldier's name. An officer from the Navy Department wrote a short note to his counterpart across town at the Interior Department, "I respectfully request per-mission to send to the hospital for the Insane, George Sympson and Anthony Castino, ordinary seamen . . . these men being reported insane by the Surgeon of the Navy Yard."[49] Although a surgeon's med-ical recommendation was curiously absent, an ill-informed bureaucracy seemingly bypassed medical advice, and when permission was granted, the Government Hospital once again received two patients without clinical records.

The Government Hospital for the Insane provided care to certain noncombatants who directly supported the military. These civilians filled critical jobs, many in the quartermaster corps. Thomas Butler had one of those jobs—until he went insane.

Sgt. John Elkins was probably confused, even though his orders were specific. Special Order Number Twenty-Six from The Headquarters of the Department of Arkansas clearly directed Sergeant Elkins to transport Thomas Butler to the Government Hospital in Washington. Sergeant Elkins dutifully complied.[50]

Sergeant Elkins probably assumed his mission would be complete after he deposited Butler at the hospital. Leaving his charge at the railroad depot, Elkins traveled alone to the hospital to finalize the transfer. The hospital surgeon was summoned upon his arrival, and Elkins explained his objective and showed the surgeon his order. The surgeon scanned the document and refused to admit Butler because he was a civilian. Sergeant Elkins was no doubt dumbfounded by the brazen contempt of the surgeon and angry about the situation he found himself in. Butler was insane and could not return to the regiment.

The Quartermaster Corps employed Thomas Butler. Butler and civilians like him were indispensable in maintaining the military supply network. Unfortunately, Butler's insanity rendered him useless.

By virtue of their critical military role, quartermaster employees were subject to military authority. As a consequence, it was naturally assumed that any injured quartermaster employee would receive military medical care. Based on that philosophy, the Arkansas Military Department turned to the Government Hospital for support with Butler's case. Regrettably the expected quid pro quo ran into an administrative logjam.

Sergeant Elkins was left with one option: Confront the Washington bureaucracy. Proceeding to the Quartermaster General's Office, "The sergeant [reported] that he cannot obtain an order for the admission of Butler into said hospital." The quartermaster's office responded with a letter to the Secretary of War. "As the Quartermaster General has no means of placing an insane man where he can be properly cared for and treated, I have the honor to request that the Secretary of War, will give an order for admission to the Insane Hospital."[51]

Sergeant Elkins probably took it for granted that this impressive appeal would overcome the hospital's resistance, but he was wrong again. "The Secretary of War has only power to give an order to admit a soldier to the Insane Asylum. The Secretary of the Interior gives orders for citizens, and there is a late act providing for such persons as the present applicant." [52] It was a maddening demonstration of priorities lost in a bureaucratic shuffle.

Sergeant Elkins's patience and persistence was eventually rewarded. The Quartermaster General's Office dutifully scribed another letter to the Interior Secretary seeking admission for Butler. With the paper chase now completed, the Government Hospital resignedly accepted the admission.

According to official government records, insanity was a rare event among soldiers and sailors. The first full year of the war counted 494 cases of insanity. As the war effort accelerated, there was a corresponding increase in cases reported. Nearly nine hundred military members fell victim to insanity in the war's second year. That was the peak year. After 1863, reported cases of insanity steadily declined.[53]

The statistics probably underestimated the real incidence. *Insanity* was a term reserved for the most blatant mental decompositions, and subtler forms of mental illness escaped that label. Perhaps "inflammation of the brain" or the much larger number of debilitating "headaches" reported in official government records concealed milder versions of insanity.

Headaches, inflammation of the brain, and insanity were official, but vague, military diagnoses and the lack of diagnostic clarity encouraged subjective interpretations. Surgeons expended great effort tabulating more than fifty thousand headaches during the war.[54] No concise definition united the victims. No doubt many mentally ill soldiers received the less stigmatizing diagnosis of headache. Surely, within that vast number a few hangovers or "mental aches" might have slipped by.

The fear of insanity was partly based on the unpredictable, and possibly infectious, nature of the disorder. Sometimes whole units were quickly overcome by a disabling mental pandemonium. Commanders and troops alike were convinced that one individual could spread the illness. Fear and ignorance were united. Examples of group insanity spread by word of mouth, and such tales were accepted with a mixture of awe, empathy, and disbelief.

The military campaign in Georgia offered all the ingredients necessary for a mass mental breakdown. Gen. William T. Sherman was unwavering in his drive to overpower Confederate resistance, and the Confederates were just as determined to destroy the enemy invader. Both sides tensely awaited the final showdown. The supreme test of wills squared off in North Georgia.[55]

Union and Confederate forces were bogged down around Marietta. The cagey rebel defenders were deeply entrenched just to the west of the city, their long line surrounding the Kennesaw Mountain. Federal forces were massing just to the east of the Confederates. Both sides anticipated a battle, although the exact location remained uncertain. Control of the high Kennesaw promontory was key to possession of the surrounding lowlands.

Unfortunately for the Federal attackers, "The Mountain itself is entirely separated from all mountain ranges, and swells up like a great bulb from the plain."[56] The Illinois officer making this assessment was impressed by the seeming invincibility of the Confederate position. Neither side seriously expected a full frontal attack on such foreboding geography, but a series of events forced Sherman to risk that foolhardy venture.

General Sherman had previously been stung by criticism faulting his cautious battlefield tactics. A public perception that he was timid was taking root, fed by aggressive newspaper reporters. Time was Sherman's other enemy. His getting bogged down in Georgia ultimately benefited Gen. Robert E. Lee's forces in Virginia. Confederate supply lines would be left intact by delay, and Federal forces couldn't be redeployed. Almost impulsively, General Sherman settled on a reckless course of action.

Sherman chose the totally unexpected and assaulted the formidable Kennesaw Mountain. Surprise would be his ally; a diversionary engagement would divide and confuse the Confederate response. Sherman allowed two days preparation for the attack. His fear of sabotage was so great that Sherman kept the battle plan a secret from staff officers on down. That turned out to be a bad idea, and it backfired.

The deception was a success of sorts. "Fire fights, picket clashes, and sudden cannonades would break into flame from point to point, then subside into sputters and die away, sporadic, inconclusive, and productive of little more than speculation. Whether off on the flanks or crouched near the critical center, men listened and wondered, unable to find a pattern to the action."[57] The Confederates monitored the situation closely but were unable to firmly grasp the enemy's intent. Confederates were confused, but Union soldiers were also left in the dark. Along the Federal lines the rumors spread like wildfire. Anxiety mounted as both sides faced the unknown.

The two days of preparation were made even more miserable by bad weather. Rain soaked the soldiers and muddied the roads. Hours before the battle began, a hot, steamy sauna-like atmosphere replaced the rain. General Sherman's plan called for a massive cannon bombardment to precede the infantry advance. For a solid hour, a furious rain of ordnance fell on Confederate positions. A brief, deafening silence followed, then, to the utter amazement of the Rebels, the Union soldiers attacked Kennesaw Mountain. A brilliant blue wave surged forward, but the crest fell far short of the Confederate defenses.

Federal soldiers, whipped by rain, intentionally misled, awed by the geography, and left mentally unprepared, were ordered to attack the Confederate center. The Confederate fusillade was murderous. As the Federal forces emerged in full view, the Confederate defenders sprayed a highly efficient fire on them. One Rebel marveled,

"They seemed to walk up and take death as coolly as if they were automatic or wooden men." A Union soldier wryly commented, "It was only necessary to expose a hand to procure a furlough."[58]

The valley of fear that Federal forces marched into claimed more than just physical casualties. Wounds suffered by this contingent were emotional, but no less effective than bullets in rendering them unfit. The injuries were self-inflicted through poor preparation. General Sherman severely minimized the value of mentally fortifying his men. Surprise had worked—against his own troops.

Soldiers of the 34th and 86th Illinois Regiments crumpled under the mental stress. Wandering aimlessly about the battlefield, clinging to their pots and pans, the confused soldiers made a tempting target. The Confederate defenders implicitly recognized the mass insanity that robbed the Union soldiers' senses, and they held their fire, refusing to take advantage of the enemy's distress. These particular Federal forces were already wounded and useless combatants.[59]

The Kennesaw Mountain experience contained a precautionary footnote. Successful preparation for combat required more than a consideration of ordnance, weather, geography, and deployment. Soldiers were not pawns to be merely moved about on an abstract field. Successful commanders entrusted their troops with knowledge, confidence, and importance of mission. Through the process, soldier's acquired a mental armor, which helped shield them from the coming horror of combat.

Many military surgeons noted that mental preparedness insulated the soldier from battle shock, and this idea was adapted to clinical practice. Open communication, predictability, and trust building were seen as helping some insane patients recover.

The blame for most cases of insanity was placed on indiscriminate recruiting, not command styles. An Annual Report of the Government Hospital complained, "It is obvious that if the recruit lacks the mental vigor and endurance necessary to receive and practice the discipline and instruction of a soldier, he will involuntarily betray both his companions and his country in the hour of battle."[60]

Lucas Hoffman was a typical patient admitted to the Government

Hospital for the Insane. His admission was prompted by the acute onset of delirium. Attempts to communicate with Hoffman were met with either silence or incoherent ramblings. Most striking was his disorientation, stemming from a global memory loss. Despite repeated entreaties, no clue emerged as to his background or factors contributing to his current debility. Hoffman voiced only one complaint—he pointed to his leg and groaned. When pressure was applied to his leg, he screamed, but careful physical diagnosis detected no obvious injury.

The patient was dangerous. Left unattended, he was vulnerable to an inadvertent injury, so efforts were made to restrict Hoffman to his room. This was a humane approach, given his infant-like tendency to wander off. Hoffman was frustrated by the limitations placed on his movements. Lacking the capacity to rationally understand the mobility restrictions, Hoffman gave direct vent to his anger. "He would frequently get out of bed and endeavor to leave the room, and on being prevented from so doing would get perfectly furious striking right and left and requiring several men to manage him."

Firm limits, patience, and a regular ward routine had a calming effect on Hoffman. His delirium never fully relented, though, in spite of the treatment. Various tonics and stimulants were administered, and, occasionally it was necessary to sedate him with opiates. Still Hoffman's behavior was unstable. An early release was not to be, because hospital physicians deemed Hoffman's mental disorder difficult to cure.[61]

Letter writing was a favorite activity of the patients, and letters were sent to staff, other patients, and family. Surviving examples provide rare insights into the troubled minds of the time. Ranging from incoherent scribbles to pseudoscholarly tomes, the musings of the insane cast light on their thinking.

Robert Rellem, a chaplain who was an inmate of the Government Hospital, was compelled to write a lengthy note to the Secretary of the Interior. Playing down the reason for his admission, the chaplain explained, "I was procured entrance here as a place of safety rather than as an Insane dangerous person." His preamble was offered as a rather deceptive introduction. The writer was clever, recognizing the incredulity that a letter from the Insane Asylum would inspire, and, by casting his admission in favorable terms, the chaplain sought to blunt that skepticism. But, as the reader descended into the letter's content, a creeping sense of the author's confusion emerged. The chaplain wrote that "strange circumstances" preceded his admission; chief among them was an unshakable belief that he was in mortal danger. To the chaplain it was inexplicable. He was convinced that he was the subject of an assassination plot. The distortion crept through his mind and controlled his behavior. He became increasingly cautious and ever more vigilant, and he began to interpret every innocent action as menacing. In response, the chaplain retreated to the relative safety of isolation. To guard further against attack, his paranoid mind demanded he abandon sleep, but eventually physical exhaustion mercifully intervened. His friends, alarmed by his social withdrawal and bizarre thinking, forced his admission to the hospital. Still misperceiving intentions, the chaplain gladly accepted an offer to hide himself from his unknown conspirators.

The chaplain's relief was temporary. Days of hypervigilance left the victim prostrate and feverish. Security had come at the expense of liberty, irritating the chaplain. "I a *loyal Man and Patriot* to my *glorious Country* . . . with my *life* and *property* on *Freedoms bleeding alter*, am guarded like a *Fellon.*"

The chaplain's repeated pleas for discharge were ignored. His confusion and paranoia simply precluded his safe return to society. As his stay lengthened and discharge became more elusive, he adopted a strident tone of belligerence in his correspondence. The Government Hospital was attacked. "I was destined to suffer . . . I *begged daily* for a *bath* . . . but *except* a little water in a slop pail . . . I was *denied.* . . . I was *compelled* to *live* in my *filthy body and clothes two weeks* . . . I *suffered* with *cold.* . . . Exercise such as I now need is *denied me.* . . . I have had *no medical care* since I *came* here."[62]

The chaplain protested further. The food was intolerable, his medical care incompetent, and his clothes ruined through inattention. To further dramatize the deplorable conditions, and advance his aim of discharge, he identified a large number of recent hospital deaths as proof of the danger his life was in. Finally, it seemed, the chaplain understood who the schemers were. Hospital personnel were now central figures in the plan to murder him. The desperate position that the chaplain's distorted mind created fueled his urgent appeals to a higher authority. The letter describing the chaplain's fate was sent to the Secretary of the Interior. It concluded with a fervent prayer. "God, and the Country call on you Sir, for investigation—for purging this *monument*." A rational letter might have swayed the reader. Unfortunately, the chaplain's sophistry betrayed his insanity.

Despite the lack of paperwork accompanying new patients, the Government Hospital for the Insane kept an abundance of records after their admission. Careful tabulation of data exposed a wealth of information. By the middle of the Civil War, nearly fifteen hundred insane individuals had been treated. About 80 percent of the patients were between twenty and forty years old. The most common diagnosis (roughly two-thirds of all new admissions) was mania. Various acute forms of mania were recognized, such as suicidal, erotic, febrile, periodical, dipsoic, cataleptic, kleptoic, and typhomania. Chronic mania was classified as simple, epileptic, paralytic, puerperal, periodical, cataleptic, homicidal, and suicidal types. The remaining one-third of the patients, in order, were diagnosed as suffering from dementia, melancholia, and monomania.[63]

Military patients accounted for nearly 85 percent of all admissions to the Government Hospital. Very few came from the Navy. Hospital personnel had a ready answer for that discrepancy. "The seaman has a more hardy and unsusceptible constitution than the landsman. In being transferred from the merchant to the naval service, he experiences few trying changes in his habits and in the moral influences about him."[64]

The administrators of the Government Hospital were proud of their success. More than half of the soldiers admitted would be listed as recovered on discharge. Many would be released from military service, and too many of them would became prey to unscrupulous

bounty recruiters and were enticed to reenlist. These gullible recruits
satisfied the greed of a nation hungry for soldiers.

Deaths at the Government Hospital were curiously included
among the count of those discharged. At the war's midpoint, 17
percent of discharges were listed as dead. Some deaths resulted from
a virulent scourge like typhoid fever. Most patients who died from
typhoid fever had been admitted with the affliction. Among
the chronically insane, a self-imposed starvation ended some
lives. "By inanition, as an assigned cause of death, is meant the non-
assimilation of food in consequence of a peculiar exhaustion of the
vital forces."[65]

The cause of insanity reflected scientific and moral speculation.
During the Civil War the number of civilian admissions to the Government Hospital declined dramatically. For some observers, this
offered proof of a moral dimension. "This evident diminution in the
relative prevalence of insanity in the District accords with the history
of the disease throughout the loyal States; and it is thought to show
that the mind of the country was raised by the war to a healthier
tension . . . than was largely the case amid the apathies and self-
indulgences of the long-continued peace and material prosperity that
preceded the great struggle."[66]

Atomistic concepts concerning the cause of insanity were popular. By naming one simple source, people believed they could avoid
the cause and, therefore, the insanity. "All weakness invites disease,
while strength repels it; and activity is a condition of strength."[67] This
straightforward homily explained why the intellectual mind was
immune from mental attack. "There are fewer dyspeptics among
scholars than among unlettered men."[68] Mental indolence was
thought to be a risk factor associated with insanity.

The scientific view of insanity studied the relationship between
cranial anatomy and behavior. "The small cranium and the heavy
inexpressive features which characterize the imbecile are often
observed on the street as well as in alms-houses . . . but we have been
much impressed by the frequency with which our attention has been

arrested by a disproportion between . . . the head and features that are usually associated with fair intellectual powers."[69]

The physicians at The Government Hospital for the Insane appeared to be struggling with an ideological conflict. It was difficult to reconcile clinical observations with the popular theory of phrenology. Phrenology had mesmerized many members of the medical community. This increasingly irreconcilable conflict led to the eventual abandonment of phrenology. The effort was not in vain, however, since the short-lived movement propelled a scientific interest in human behavior.

The Civil War forced the nation to grudgingly recognize the emotional cost of the war. Physicians confronted disorders that had no other logical explanation. Special hospitals, such as Turner's Lane and The Government Hospital for the Insane, were clinical laboratories that launched the beginnings of a new medical revolution, where mind and body were thought of as united. As knowledge of mental illness very slowly migrated from a moral etiology to a medical basis, the interface with the legal system changed. Soldiers clearly identified as mentally ill were medically evacuated to a hospital, sometimes following serious misconduct. There were very few insanity trials, and those that were recorded involved arguable evidence of mental illness or a misguided court-martial imposing punishment instead of recommending treatment.

CHAPTER SEVEN

LESSONS LEARNED

The war was over, but victory remained elusive. Forceful reunification had succeeded in preserving territorial integrity, but a vast yawning chasm otherwise separated the North and the South. Distrust, bitterness, sadness, retribution, and a myriad of similar emotions kept the former antagonists warily apart. Families turned inward, mourning their losses. Vast cemeteries were a constant reminder of the war's cost. After the South capitulated, both armies demobilized. Soldiers returned home, many bearing emotional and physical scars. Four years of frenzied military growth came to an abrupt end, and America settled into an uneasy peace.

Long after the last bullet was fired, the impact of the Civil War continued. A new army replaced the old. The new army recruited only veterans, its members the maimed survivors of the Civil War. Every city in the nation contributed men to this new army. They were the emotional and physical casualties of the late war. Once again, America was challenged to support her men in battle. The enemy was pain, suffering, and lingering disability. Valuable lessons were learned about this enemy during the Civil War—and were applied in the aftermath of the old struggle, to aid victims in their new fight. William

A. Hammond, a former military surgeon general who favored punishment of insanity when coupled with misconduct, personified one view. The progressive approach, sponsored by superintendents of America's insane asylums, fought for compassion. This group of influential physician administrators sought remission of criminal prosecution to advance treatment of the insane.

A few months before General Robert E. Lee surrendered his command at Appomattox County Courthouse, Dr. John Gray was attending a conference, where the doctor recounted several examples of inhumane treatment of mentally ill soldiers. His audience was made up of members of the Association of Medical Superintendents of the American Institutions for the Insane. There were lessons to be learned, and Dr. Gray was an eager teacher.[1]

Soldiers gripped by madness were a disturbing prospect for Civil War surgeons. Insanity was poorly understood, at best conceptualized as a moral weakness. Even worse, it was stubbornly resistant to traditional medical interventions. A fortunate few made it safely through evacuation channels to asylums or hospitals, but an untold number were simply released from their unit—abandoned to the mercy of strangers and fate.

Dr. Gray and his like-minded colleagues abhorred the negligent treatment of the insane, and they petitioned the Army Surgeon General for relief. Their pointed questions were a clearly calculated ploy to embarrass—and force change. Among the criticisms leveled as questions by Gray were: Why were mentally ill soldiers abandoned by the military? Why were insane soldiers prosecuted for misconduct? and Why had the military failed to establish arrangements with state asylums for treatment?

The complaints prompted a swift response. The Army Surgeon General issued an order after reviewing the doctor's letter: Henceforth state hospital superintendents were empowered to certify insanity. Once a patient was declared insane by the superintendent, he was prevented from being prosecuted. The practical effect of such enlightened treatment of the mentally ill was limited, however, as most field surgeons ignored the order.

One legacy of Civil War experience was a drive to remove insane citizens from public view. State asylums swelled, whether insane soldiers arrived by accident or were purposely directed to them. A number of factors contributed to the growth of state mental asylums. For years, lurid tales of inhumane treatment of the mentally ill had bombarded the public. As America slowly became more industrial and urbanized, the poor insane congregated in the larger cities. Almshouses and jails were poorly equipped to handle the mentally ill. Another influence was military demobilization. Johnny was coming home—disabled and distraught.

At the beginning of the Civil War, roughly 8,500 patients resided in mental asylums. Five years later, America's population had grown by 2 percent, and the number of insane citizens doubled in the same time span. Every ten years through the remainder of the nineteenth century, the population of asylum patients repeatedly doubled. The upward trend continued for another fifty years. By that time, hospitals were groaning under the weight of a bloated census. Public funding declined, and many institutions became human warehouses, boxing the insane firmly inside.[2]

The Civil War accelerated the trend toward institutional care of the mentally ill. Optimism was the fuel driving the philosophy. Advocates of institutionalization compared almshouses, jails, and homelessness, and they chose the clearly superior paternalistic approach of hospital care. Hospitals offered compassionate treatment, security, and a predictable environment. Many years later, that contract was broken. Large state hospitals lost the trust of the public and they were dismantled. Freed from the institutions, the mentally ill were again aimlessly congregating in urban areas.

The Civil War boosted interest in medical-legal matters, which was a decidedly two-edged sword. Spearheading the controversy was William Hammond, who had been appointed Surgeon General early in the war. Hammond possessed a mountainous ego, and, had he harnessed that energy solely to the task of organizing the medical department, his legacy would have been untarnished. To his immense credit, Hammond tackled a hotbed of medical incompetence. Overcoming the resistance of an entrenched bureaucracy guaranteed fireworks. Hammond's chief failing was indiscriminate criticism. He immediately locked horns with his boss, Secretary of War Edwin M. Stanton. It was a bitter, protracted power struggle, which Hammond was destined to lose.[3]

Hammond and Stanton engaged in subterranean, backdoor character assaults of the worst type. Stanton clearly had the advantage, since he had the levers of power and was willingly to use them. Stanton quietly aligned the military legal system against Hammond. Then in a dramatic gesture, he relieved Hammond of his position in 1863. The Surgeon General was incensed. Hammond was a fighter, and, despite the dismissal, he flung stinging accusations at Stanton, the gist of which was Stanton's unrelenting interference in reforming the medical department. Stanton cited mismanagement as the reason for relieving Hammond. That charge chafed Hammond, and he repeatedly demanded a public trial, which Stanton willingly obliged.

Hammond's court-martial was sensational. Charges and countercharges flew fast and thick. The outcome, despite the drama, was inevitable: Hammond was convicted. Stanton punished both Hammond and the military legal system. Both were severely bruised by escalating a personality clash into criminal misconduct.

Long before his celebrated court-martial in 1864, William Hammond had a deep interest in medical jurisprudence. Far from dampening his enthusiasm, the court-martial seemed to accelerate his interest. Hammond had a personality that craved controversy. Following the war, Hammond returned to clinical practice. The emerging field of neurology was his passion. It was the perfect platform from which to launch himself as an expert in insanity. He published widely and testified everywhere.

Hammond's concept of insanity was shaped by his military background, pugnacious attitude, and clinical experience. What galled his growing bastion of opponents was the appearance of ethical impropriety. Hammond's expert testimony on diverse medical-legal issues was contradictory. The only theme unifying his testimony was an apparent zeal to win. His exorbitant fees—sometimes seemingly tied to a favorable outcome—damaged his reputation.

Hammond grew increasingly strained with his prime rivals—the superintendents of America's asylums. The basis of the disagreement was a quirky theory Hammond supported. Eschewing compassion for the mentally deranged, Hammond repeatedly testified that insanity merited punishment. The enlightened view, held by the superintendents, insisted that severe mental illness vitiated criminal responsibility. According to the superintendents, the insane belonged in hospitals not prisons. The acrimonious philosophical debate was fused with an intense dislike of Hammond.

Hammond was on the brink of recreating another Stanton-like conflict with Eugene Grissom, an asylum superintendent. It was a devastating verbal assault propelled by Grissom's publication of "True and False Experts," which savagely criticized Hammond, that caused the clash.[4]

Dr. Grissom was a learned man who possessed both medical and legal degrees. His administrative talent had been recognized by a promotion to superintendent of the North Carolina Insane Asylum. "True and False Experts" was partially the culmination of years of frustrations in dealing with the legal management of the criminally insane. Grissom read his venal attack before the Association of American Superintendents meeting in Washington, D.C. It was a receptive audience. Like a train slowly gathering speed, Grissom began his journey with a historical review.

"There was a period in history, not so very remote, when the recognition of insanity as the result of physical disease had not dawned upon wakening humanity and civilization." In the most poetic language, Dr. Grissom reminded the audience that only "a hundred and twenty years ago, when Christendom witnessed the tortures of Robert François Damiens, who in a maniacal paroxysm, wounded Louis XV. The merciful law burned his hand, tore his flesh with red-hot pincers, poured melted lead and sulphur into the wounds, and tore him apart with four horses, after many efforts, amid the jokes of the pitiful insane wretch."[5]

Grissom pointed with pride to the scientific advances that had taken place in the century since that dreadful event transpired. Armed with new knowledge, medical doctors had battled ignorance. Progress was measured in terms of more humane judicial dispositions of the insane, although Grissom admitted it remained an uphill struggle. Public opinion, when expressed by a jury, was dominated by a tendency to fear mental illness and punish misconduct. Dr. Grissom, along with his fellow asylum superintendents, was a leader in the effort to shape a more compassionate view of the insane. Their energies were often expended in lobbying legislators for new insane asylums and statutory remedies for the mentally ill. The public largely ignored these endeavors.

Unfortunately for Dr. Grissom, not all physicians agreed with his philosophic approach to the insane. Disagreement erupted in the most violent fashion—in the courtrooms of America. The asylum superintendents feared a public debate. They were deeply mistrustful of the lay citizenry, considering them wholly inept at judging insanity. The superintendents espoused a different judicial forum to weigh insanity: They wanted to replace the lay jury with scientific experts. The same imperious attitude that dismissed the intelligence of an average citizen was extended to anyone who disagreed with their assessment. A society of neurologists constantly challenged the asylum superintendents. The neurologists, among them Dr. Hammond, were opposed to the institution-building superintendents. Hammond favored moral accountability—whether the individual was insane or not. "If you do not punish the madman, you hold out a premium for every man would calculate that he would be fortunate enough to escape by someone proving that he was mad." Hammond endorsed this clearly defensible judicial opinion. In doing so, he ran counter to esteemed physicians like Dr. Gray, who believed "that no case of moral imbecility exists without some deprivation of intellect and reason."[6]

Hammond was not shy, and he rendered his medical opinion frequently. His position was more than irksome. It threatened the superintendents' hegemony in two areas: the medical jurisprudence of insanity and the future of institutional care for the mentally ill. Hammond was fast becoming a leper in need of isolation.

Dr. Grissom and the venerable Dr. Gray considered themselves "True Experts," while Dr. Hammond was vilified as a "False Expert." Aside from disagreeing with a "True Expert," the chief distinction of the "False Expert" was a record of testifying in a contradictory manner. It was a silly criticism made more ludicrous by Grissom's commentary on the adversarial procedure of a criminal trial. "One of the primary demands, therefore, on the witness-stand, is a classification from the expert, of the forms of insanity . . . and once obtained, the forensic struggle is made to show that the expert has failed when drawing his lines, 'to divide a hair twixt south and south-west side', or to triumphantly show that the accused may not belong to the special division . . . the expert may have unwarily assigned him."[7]

Dr. Grissom completely discounted contradictory testimony as a byproduct of the trial process or the imprecise state of medical diagnosis. His attack of Hammond on these charges was weakened by that oversight. Nonetheless, Hammond was guilty of inconsistent testimony at times. That complaint served chiefly as a means to attack the real target: Hammond's insistence that moral accountability accompanied all behavior, whether insane or not.

Grissom was less than halfway through his medical presentation when he unleashed his most critical verbal volley. "Is it true that the former honorable record of testimony has been recently darkened by the conduct of men more wicked than the victims whom they judged . . . and holding up the just claims of medical skill to the scorn of mankind?"[8]

The verbal flogging of Hammond was punishing. Hammond's prior testimony was dredged up, contradictions were cited as proof of his malevolence, and he was summarily judged. "Now at last we shudder as we recognize that the false expert is no man at all, but a moral monster, whose baleful eyes glare with delusive light; whose bowels are but bags of gold, to feed which, spider-like, he casts his loathsome arms about a helpless prey."[9]

Dr. Hammond responded to the vitriolic words with his own

venom. In letters made public, Hammond sniped, "A distempered and snarling cur has nobler mental and moral qualities than you . . . the foul bird that defecates in its own nest is less odious." Both sides sacrificed a reasoned debate to settle personal vendettas.[10]

The seeds of this great medical-legal controversy were sown during the Civil War. Substantive advancements were limited by the distraction of fighting a war. Madness, malingering, and malfeasance received cursory attention. Punishment remained de rigueur. Occasionally, as with Pvt. Lorenzo Stewart of New York, that automatic reflex was suspended. In the brief period allotted for an in-depth criminal defense, medical experts like Dr. Gray had an opportunity to soften the harshness of military justice. Private Stewart was not a recipient of such mercy—or so he thought. "Upon a review of the whole testimony, my opinion of the prisoner is, that he has a certain moral infirmity, not amounting to insanity; that he is an eccentric, peculiar, and in some respects, a weak man, but in no proper sense of the word, an insane man. He exhibits an instance of a condition of mind nearly allied to insanity, yet not within the borders of absolute mental alienation." With those words, Dr. Gray sealed Private Stewart's fate.[11]

Private Stewart shared a cell with Charles Varion in the Chemung County Jail, in Elmira, New York. Varion was awaiting trial for forgery. Stewart's section of the cell was neatly decorated with pictures. He had a small desk from which he wrote his public correspondence. His only other possessions, aside from personal articles, were some books. A certain degree of freedom was permitted the inmates until late evening, at which time, all cells were locked. At some point, the whispers exchanged between Stewart and Varion turned toward escape. Of the pair, Stewart was surely the motivated partner. He also had skill on his side. Somehow, Stewart always finagled his way out of harm's way, and with Varion's help, this time he did it again.

The *Elmira Daily Gazette* reported the exploits of Stewart for the last time on January 12, 1865. The bold headline shouted, "Great Jail Outbreak—Escape of Seven Prisoners from Chemung County Jail by Tunneling—Stewart Among the Number."[12]

Embarrassed jail officials launched an immediate investigation. Apparently, Stewart and his cohort had stolen away sometime between evening lockdown and breakfast call—an interval approaching eleven hours. The sheriff soon came across the tunnel. "A hole was discovered . . . which was found to extend to the outside. . . . One of the boards had been taken up, and a hole cut through about six inches of hard cement to the depth of about two feet and a half, then tunneling was commenced eastward . . . for nearly twenty feet . . . coming up just outside the jail walls." About the only item of value Stewart left behind was a letter richly bragging about his successful escape. Although an aggressive effort was made to recapture Stewart, it failed, and he remained free.

Thirteen years would pass before the saga of Lorenzo Stewart came to a close. His wife, family, friends, and political associates worked tirelessly to clear his name. Their activities culminated in President Rutherford B. Hayes requesting documentary evidence supporting a pardon. From his home in Vermont, LeRoy Shear, alias Lorenzo Stewart, prepared his "True Statement."

The "True Statement" was a respectful plea. "Your Excellency told me to send you, by Express, my statement of the matter." Testimonial letters from local politicians were appended. "Exhibit A" was a brief summary of a discussion purportedly held between President Lincoln and Senator Ira Harris. "President Lincoln said to Hon. Ira Harris that he felt I never intended to do what I did and . . . he would send me a pardon." President Hayes granted the pardon. In late March 1878 Stewart received his unconditional freedom.[13]

America entered the Civil War as a nation divided. With the South's capitulation, a long, painful rapprochement began. The national healing process demanded that lessons be learned, as if to justify the lives lost. In the years following the war, a dimly outlined consensus could be seen favoring compassion, tolerance, and respect for the mentally ill who appeared before a legal authority. The medical and legal professions, with help from enlightened politicians and citizen advocates, preached these virtues. Their success resurrected a moribund military medical service, pressured leaders to recognize inequities in military law, and supported innovative solutions to complex problems.

Madness, Malingering, and Malfeasance: Lorenzo Stewart's case epitomized the intersection of these complex behaviors. His experience, and that of countless others, helped shape the future face of medical jurisprudence in America.

ENDNOTES

ENDNOTES TO INTRODUCTION

1. George Worthington Adams, *Doctors in Blue: The Medical History of the Union Army in the Civil War* (Dayton, OH: Press of Morningside, 1985), 76.

2. Thomas Maeder, *Crime and Madness: The Origins and Evolutions of the Insanity Defense* (New York: Harper and Row, 1985), 23–35.

3. Maeder, *Crime and Madness*, 28–29.

4. Maeder, *Crime and Madness*, 10.

5. Maeder, *Crime and Madness*, 26.

6. Maeder, *Crime and Madness*, 28–29.

7. Maeder, *Crime and Madness*, 30.

8. Maeder, *Crime and Madness*, 22–23.

9. James C. Mohr, *Doctors and the Law: Medical Jurisprudence in Nineteenth-Century America* (New York: Oxford University Press, 1993), 160.

10. William Winthrop, *Military Law and Precedents* (Washington, DC: War Department, Office of Adjutant General, 1886), 953–960. William Winthrop was an attorney who entered the Union

Army in April 1861. In the preface to the first edition, Winthrop describes his motivation to author this text: "In view of the absence and want of a comprehensive treatise and the science of Military Law, it has been for some year[s] the purpose of the author . . . to attempt to supply such want with a work." Colonel Winthrop authored the authoritative legal treatise covering the Civil War.

11. Winthrop, *Military Law and Precedents,* 961–971.

12. Winthrop, *Military Law and Precedents,* 23.

13. Winthrop, *Military Law and Precedents,* 23.

14. Bvt. Lieut. Colonel S. V. Benét, *A Treatise on Military Law and the Practice of the Courts-Martial* (New York: D. Van Nostrand, 1868), 405. Benét continuously updated his *Treatise on Military Law* throughout the Civil War. His efforts apparently began early in 1862 and led to successive revised editions. Benét analyzed opinions issued by the War Department, Judge Advocate of the Army, and selected courts-martial.

15. Benét, *Treatise on Military Law,* 409.

16. Benét, *Treatise on Military Law,* 406.

17. Benét, *Treatise on Military Law,* 407.

18. Benét, *Treatise on Military Law,* 407.

19. Benét, *Treatise on Military Law,* 411.

20. Benét, *Treatise on Military Law,* 409.

21. Benét, *Treatise on Military Law,* 409.

22. Maj. Gen. George B. Davis, *A Treatise on the Military Law of the United States: Together with the Practice and Procedure of the Courts-Martial and Other Military Tribunals* (New York: John Wiley and Sons, 1915) 124–131.

23. Benét, *Treatise on Military Law,* 413.

ENDNOTES TO CHAPTER ONE

1. National Archives. J.A.G. Records LL1431. *Elmira Daily Gazette,* 1 Nov. 1863.

2. National Archives. J.A.G. Records LL1431. "General Court-Martial," *Elmira Daily Gazette,* 2 Dec. 1863.

3. J.A.G. Records LL1431. *Elmira Daily Gazette,* 1 Nov. 1863.
4. National Archives. J.A.G. Records LL1431. Transcript of the Special Court of Inquiry, April-May 1864: 18–19.
5. J.A.G. Records LL1431. Special Court of Inquiry, 20–21.
6. J.A.G. Records LL1431. *Elmira Daily Gazette,* 1 Nov. 1863.
7. National Archives. J.A.G. Records LL1431. "The Stewart Desertion and Murder Case," *Elmira Daily Gazette,* 23 Dec. 1863.
8. J.A.G. Records LL1431. *Elmira Daily Gazette,* 23 Dec. 1863.
9. J.A.G. Records LL1431. *Elmira Daily Gazette,* 23 Dec. 1863.
10. J.A.G. Records LL1431. *Elmira Daily Gazette,* 23 Dec. 1863.
11. J.A.G. Records LL1431. "All Hopes Gone," *Elmira Daily Gazette,* 21 Apr. 1864.
12. National Archives. J.A.G. Records LL1431. E. D. Townsend, Assistant Adjutant General. "To Major General Dix," 21 Apr. 1864. Copy of a Telegram.
13. National Archives. J.A.G. Records LL1431. A letter from Lorenzo C. Stewart while incarcerated in Chemung County Jail, dated 20 April 1864, Elmira, NY.
14. National Archives. J.A.G. Records LL1431. *Elmira Daily Gazette,* 21 Apr. 1864.
15. National Archives. J.A.G. Records LL1431. *Elmira Daily Gazette,* 21 Apr. 1864.
16. National Archives. J.A.G. Records LL1431. Letter from Private Stewart to President Abraham Lincoln from Chemung County Jail, 30 Mar. 1864.
17. National Archives. J.A.G. Records LL1431. "Suspension of Stewart's Sentence," *Elmira Daily Gazette,* 24 Apr. 1864.
18. National Archives. J.A.G. Records LL1431. "Suspension of Stewart's Sentence," *Elmira Daily Gazette,* 24 Apr. 1864.
19. National Archives. J.A.G. Records LL1431. Letter from President Abraham Lincoln to Dr. John P. Gray, Utica, NY. In the matter of the inquiry into the mental condition of Lorenzo C. Stewart. From the Executive Mansion, Washington, DC, 25 Apr. 1864. Dr. John P. Gray was Superintendent of the State Lunatic Asylum, Utica, NY.

20. John P. Gray, "Case of Lorenzo C. Stewart," *American Journal of Insanity* (Jan. 1865): 18–21.
21. National Archives. J.A.G. Records LL1431. Transcript Special Court of Inquiry, 18.
22. National Archives. J.A.G. Records LL1431. Transcript Special Court of Inquiry, 18–21.
23. National Archives. J.A.G. Records LL1431. Transcript Special Court of Inquiry, 20.
24. National Archives. J.A.G. Records LL1431. Transcript Special Court of Inquiry, 20.
25. National Archives. J.A.G. Records LL1431. Transcript Special Court of Inquiry, 129–135.
26. National Archives. J.A.G. Records LL1431. Transcript Special Court of Inquiry, 245–259.
27. National Archives. J.A.G. Records LL1431. Transcript Special Court of Inquiry, 104.
28. National Archives. J.A.G. Records LL1431. Transcript Special Court of Inquiry, 80.
29. National Archives. J.A.G. Records LL1431. Transcript Special Court of Inquiry, 68.
30. Gray 18–21.
31. National Archives. J.A.G. Records LL1431. Letter from Lorenzo C. Stewart while incarcerated in Chemung County Jail, dated 20 April 1864, Elmira, NY.
32. Isaac Ray, *A Treatise on the Medical Jurisprudence of Insanity* (Cambridge, MA: The Belknap Press of Harvard University Press, 1962), x–xii.

ENDNOTES TO CHAPTER TWO

1. John Bartlett, *Familiar Quotations*, sixteenth ed. (Boston: Little, Brown and Company, 1992), 100. Publilius Syrus authored a vast collection of maxims. These words of wisdom were collected in more than 1,000 adages. This particular quote was number 750.
2. National Archives. *RG 94. Records of the Adjutant General's*

Office; hereinafter cited as *RG 94.* M1523, "Proceedings of U.S. Army Courts-Martial and Military Commissions of Union Soldiers Executed by U.S. Military Authorities, 1861–1866."

3. Charles A. Humphreys, *Field, Camp, Hospital and Prison in the Civil War, 1863–1865* (Freeport, NY: Books for Libraries Press, 1971), 19.

4. Humphreys, *Field, Camp, Hospital and Prison,* 19.

5. Humphreys, *Field, Camp, Hospital and Prison,* 20.

6. Humphreys, *Field, Camp, Hospital and Prison,* 20–21.

7. *RG 94.* "List of U.S. Soldiers Executed by United States Military Authorities During the Late War."

8. *RG 94.* "List of U.S. Soldiers Executed by United States Military Authorities During the Late War."

9. Bvt. Lieut. Colonel S. V. Benét, *A Treatise on Military Law and the Practice of the Courts-Martial* (New York: D. Van Nostrand, 1868), 413.

10. Benét, *A Treatise on Military Law,* 395–396.

11. John D. Billings, *Hardtack and Coffee or the Unwritten Story of Army Life* (Boston: George M. Smith, 1887), 157–159.

12. John M. Greiner, Janet L. Coryell, and James R. Smither, eds., *A Surgeon's Civil War: The Letters and Diary of Daniel M. Holt, M.D.* (Kent, OH: Kent State University Press, 1994), 131.

13. Billings, *Hardtack and Coffee,* 161.

14. Bell Irvin Wiley, *The Life of Billy Yank: The Common Soldier of the Union* (Indianapolis: Bobbs-Merrill, 1952), 207.

15. James I. Robertson, "Military Executions," *Civil War Times Illustrated,* 2 (1966): 38–39.

16. *RG 94.* Case of William Lynch, file no. 2533, roll no. 3. Also see General Court-Martial Order 35, Army of the Potomac, 1864.

17. *RG 94.* "List of U.S. Soldiers Executed by United States Military Authorities During the Late War."

18. Robertson, "Military Executions," 36.

19. Billings, *Hardtack and Coffee,* 161.

20. *RG 94.* Case of George W. McDonald, file no. LL2430, roll no. 3. Also see General Orders 74, Middle Department, 1864.

21. *RG 94*. Case of Charles Sperry, file no. NN2427, roll no. 7. Also see General Orders 31, Department of Washington, 1865.
22. *RG 94*. Case of James Preble, file no. MM1774, roll no. 7. Also see General Orders 22, Department of North Carolina, 1865.
23. *RG 94*. Case of Michael Wert, file no. LL2924, roll no. 8. Also see General Court-Martial Orders 1, Army of the Potomac, 1865.
24. *RG 94*. Case of Henry Hamilton, file no. LL2628, roll no. 2. Also see General Orders 132, Department of the Gulf, 1864.
25. Thomas P. Lowry, *Don't Shoot That Boy!: Abraham Lincoln and Military Justice* (Mason City, IA: Savas Publishing, 1999), v–22.
26. R. A. Brock, ed. *Southern Historical Society Papers,* vol. 21 (Richmond, VA: Broad Foot Publishing, 1990), 326–337.
27. John P. Gray, "The Case of Dr. David M. Wright, for the Murder of Lieutenant Sanborn—Plea, Insanity," *American Journal of Insanity* 20 (1864): 286. Dr. John P. Gray was the Superintendent of the New York State Lunatic Asylum, the same physician who examined Private Lorenzo Stewart.
28. Brock, *Southern Historical Society Papers,* 333–334.
29. Arthur G. Sharp, "Men of Peace," *Civil War Times Illustrated,* 21, 4 (June 1982): 30–37.

ENDNOTES TO CHAPTER THREE

1. General Order 122, Department of Missouri, 1864.
2. General Order 153, Department of Missouri, 1864.
3. General Order 153, Department of Missouri, 1864.
4. General Order 153, Department of Missouri, 1864.
5. General Order 153, Department of Missouri, 1864.
6. Bvt. Lieut. Colonel S. V. Benét, *A Treatise on Military Law and the Practice of Courts-Martial* (New York: D. Van Nostrand, 1868), 401.
7. Benét, *A Treatise on Military Law,* 271–272.
8. Benét, *A Treatise on Military Law,* 272–273.
9. General Orders 7, War Department, 1856.
10. General Orders 53, 98, Army of the Potomac, 1862.

11. General Court-Martial Orders 13, Department of Missouri, 1882.

12. General Orders 48, Department of Virginia, 1864.

13. General Orders 45, Department of the Pacific, 1863.

14. Col. William Winthrop, *Military Law and Precedents* (Washington, DC: Government Printing Office, 1920), 340.

15. General Orders 5, Department of the Pacific, 1864.

16. Winthrop, *Military Law and Precedents,* 718.

17. *RG 94.* Case of James Weaver, alias N. E. Baker, file no. OO316, roll no. 8. Also see General Orders 12, Army of the Potomac, 1865.

18. *RG 94.* Case of Henry Holt, file no. MM1427, roll no. 2. Also see General Orders 43, Department of Virginia and North Carolina, 1864.

19. *RG 94.* Case of Larkin Ray, file no. NN3261, roll no. 7. Also see General Orders 178, Department of the Gulf, 1864.

20. *RG 94.* Case of Darius Philbrooks, file no. II953, roll no. 7. Also see General Orders 25, Department of New Mexico, 1862.

21. *Medical and Surgical History of the War of the Rebellion,* vol. 1, pt. 3 (Washington, DC: Government Printing Office, 1888).

22. *Medical and Surgical History of the War of the Rebellion,* vol. 1, pt. 3.

23. Bell Irvin Wiley, *The Life of Billy Yank: The Common Soldier of the Union* (Indianapolis: Bobbs-Merrill, 1952) 296–312.

24. Wiley, *The Life of Billy Yank,* 230–231.

25. Bell I. Wiley, "The Common Soldier of the Civil War," *Civil War Times Illustrated* (Special Issue, 1973), 48.

26. John D. Billings, *Hardtack and Coffee or the Unwritten Story of Army Life* (Boston: George M. Smith, 1887), 145.

27. General Orders 30, Department of Missouri, 1864.

28. Major-General George B. Davis, *A Treatise on the Military Law of the United States* (New York: John Wiley and Sons, 1915), 126.

29. Davis, *A Treatise on the Military Law,* 127.

30. General Orders 37, Middle Department, 1864.

31. Isaac Ray, *A Treatise on the Medical Jurisprudence of Insanity*

(Cambridge, MA: The Belknap Press of Harvard University Press, 1962), x–xii.

32. Ray, *A Treatise on the Medical Jurisprudence of Insanity,* x–xii.
33. Ray, *A Treatise on the Medical Jurisprudence of Insanity,* 312–314.
34. Ray, *A Treatise on the Medical Jurisprudence of Insanity,* 314.
35. Ray, *A Treatise on the Medical Jurisprudence of Insanity,* 309–310.
36. Ray, *A Treatise on the Medical Jurisprudence of Insanity,* 324.
37. Stanley L. Swart, "The Military Examination Board in the Civil War: A Case Study," *Civil War History* vol. 16, 3 (Sept. 1970): 228.
38. Swart, "The Military Examination Board in the Civil War," 231.
39. Wiley, *Life of Billy Yank,* 130.
40. Wiley, *Life of Billy Yank,* 130–131.
41. George Worthington Adams, *Doctors in Blue: The Medical History of the Union Army in the Civil War* (Dayton, OH: Press of Morningside, 1985), 55.
42. General Orders 126, Department of Missouri, 1864.
43. General Orders 101, Department of Missouri, 1864.
44. General Orders 80, Department of Missouri, 1864.

ENDNOTES TO CHAPTER FOUR

1. John D. Billings, *Hardtack and Coffee or the Unwritten Story of Army Life* (Boston: George M. Smith, 1887), 162.
2. *RG 48.* Department of the Interior. Rules and Regulations of the United States Jail, 1857.
3. *RG 48.* Department of the Interior. Rules and Regulations of the United States Jail, 1857.
4. *RG 48.* Department of the Interior. Correspondence between Dr. Duhamel and the Secretary of the Interior, 1867.
5. *RG 48.* Department of the Interior. Report of the Warden of the Jail, Nov. 1865.
6. *RG 48.* Department of the Interior. Report of the Warden from the U.S. Jail, July 1865.
7. *RG 48.* Department of the Interior. Rules and Regulations, House of Refuge, Baltimore, MD.

8. *RG 48.* Department of the Interior. Report of the Warden from the U.S. Jail, Nov. 1865.

9. *RG 48.* Department of the Interior. Letter and Reward Poster from an Inspector at the U.S. Jail to the Secretary of the Interior, 1860.

10. *RG 48.* Department of the Interior. Jail Record Books, 1865.

11. *RG 48.* Department of the Interior. U.S. Jail Docket, 1863.

12. *RG 48.* Department of the Interior. U.S. Jail Docket, 1865.

13. *RG 48.* Department of the Interior. U.S. Jail Docket, 1863.

14. *RG 48.* Department of the Interior. Record Book, 1862.

15. *RG 48.* Department of the Interior. Report of the Warden of the Jail, Nov. 1865.

ENDNOTES TO CHAPTER FIVE

1. William Winthrop, *Military Law and Precedents,* 2nd ed. rev. and enl. (Washington: Government Printing Office, 1920), 730.

2. Eugene Murdock, *Patriotism Limited 1862–1865: The Civil War Draft and the Bounty System* (Kent, OH: Kent University Press, 1967), chapter 5.

3. Eugene C. Murdock, "Pity the Poor Surgeon," *Civil War History,* vol. 16, 1 (March 1970): 26.

4. Murdock, "Pity," 22.

5. Murdock, "Pity," 23.

6. Murdock, "Pity," 22–23.

7. John D. Billings, *Hardtack and Coffee or the Unwritten Story of Army Life* (Boston: George M. Smith and Company, 1887), 100.

8. Billings, *Hardtack and Coffee,* 100.

9. Murdock, "Pity," 29.

10. Murdock, "Pity," 29.

11. Murdock, "Pity," 29.

12. Murdock, "Pity," 29–30.

13. Murdock, "Pity," 30.

14. Allen D. Spiegel and Florence Kavaler, "Abraham Lincoln, Medical Jurisprudence, and Chloroform—Induced Insanity in an 1857 Murder Trial," *Caduceus* (Winter 1994): 145–160.

15. Murdock, "Pity," 31.

16. Thomas P. Lowry, M.D., *Tarnished Eagles: The Courts-Martial of Fifty Union Colonels and Lieutenant Colonels* (Mechanicsburg, PA: Stackpole Books, 1997).

17. Stanley L. Swart, "The Military Examination Board in the Civil War: A Case Study," *Civil War History,* vol. 16, 3 (Sept. 1970): 228.

18. Swart, "The Military Examination Board in the Civil War," 239.

19. Swart, "The Military Examination Board in the Civil War," 233–237.

20. Swart, "The Military Examination Board in the Civil War," 243–244.

21. Bruce Catton, *Bruce Catton's Civil War: Three Volumes in One* (New York: Fairfax Press, 1984), 586.

22. Billings, *Hardtack and Coffee,* 95.

23. Leander Stillwell, *The Story of a Common Soldier of Army Life in the Civil War: 1861–1865,* 2nd ed. (Erie, KS: Franklin Hudson Publishing, 1920), 119–120.

24. Gerald F. Linderman, *Embattled Courage: The Experience of Combat in the American Civil War* (New York: Free Press, 1987), 156–168.

25. Bell Irvin Wiley, *The Life of Billy Yank: The Common Soldier of the Union* (Indianapolis: Bobbs-Merril, 1952), 289–291.

26. Wiley, *Life of Billy Yank,* 291.

27. Catton, *Bruce Catton's Civil War,* 284.

28. Eugene C. Murdock, "Pity the Poor Surgeon," *Civil War History,* vol. 16 1 (March 1930), 32.

29. J. M. Da Costa, M.D., "On Irritable Heart: A Clinical Study of a Form of Functional Cardiac Disorder and Its Consequences," *The American Journal of the Medical Sciences,* 121 (Jan. 1871): 36–37.

30. Albert Castel, ed., "Malingering: 'Many . . . Diseases Are . . . Feigned.,'" *Civil War Times Illustrated* 16, 5 (Aug. 1977): 29.

31. Castel, "Malingering," 30.

32. Castel, "Malingering," 29.

33. Castel, "Malingering," 30.

34. Castel, "Malingering," 32.

35. Castel, "Malingering," 32.

36. Winthrop, *Military Law and Precedents,* 959.

37. Winthrop, *Military Law and Precedents,* 960.

38. Winthrop, *Military Law and Precedents,* 730–731.

39. Winthrop, *Military Law and Precedents,* 723.

40. General Orders 33, Department of Ohio, 1863.

41. General Orders 33, Department of Ohio, 1863.

42. General Orders 37, Middle Department, 1864.

43. General Court-Martial Orders 29, Department of Missouri, 1869.

ENDNOTES TO CHAPTER SIX

1. General Orders 13, Northern Department, 1864.

2. General Court-Martial Orders 39, Department of Missouri, 1868.

3. William Winthrop, *Military Law and Precedents* (Washington DC: War Department, Office of Adjutant General, 1886), 621.

4. R. Gregory Lande and David Armitage, eds., *Principles and Practice of Military Forensic Psychiatry* (Springfield, IL: Charles C. Thomas, 1997), 9.

5. General Orders 96, Department of New Mexico, 1862.

6. Lande and Armitage, *Principles and Practice,* 9.

7. General Orders 10, Department of the Gulf, 1866.

8. General Orders 10, Department of the Gulf, 1866.

9. General Orders 91, Army of the Potomac, 1863.

10. General Orders 91, Army of the Potomac, 1863.

11. General Orders 91, Army of the Potomac, 1863.

12. General Orders 91, Army of the Potomac, 1863.

13. General Orders 54, Department of the Pacific, 1864.

14. General Orders 54, Department of the Pacific, 1864.

15. General Orders 54, Department of the Pacific, 1864.

16. General Orders 54, Department of the Pacific, 1864.

17. Thomas P. Lowry, M.D. and Jack D. Walsh, M.D., *Tarnished Scalpels: The Court-Martials of Fifty Union Surgeons* (Mechanicsburg, PA: Stackpole Books, 2000), xvii–xxix.

18. Bell Irvin Wiley, *The Life of Billy Yank: The Common Soldier of the Union* (Indianapolis: Bobbs-Merrill, 1952), 141–151.

19. Page Smith, *Trial by Fire: A People's History of the Civil War and Reconstruction* (New York: McGraw-Hill, 1982), 393–398.

20. Wiley, *The Life of Billy Yank*, 290.

21. Wiley, *The Life of Billy Yank*, 292.

22. *The Medical and Surgical History of the War of the Rebellion*, Vol. 1, pt. 3 (Washington, DC: Government Printing Office, 1888), 884–886.

23. *The Medical and Surgical History of the War of the Rebellion*, vol. 1, pt. 3 (Washington, DC: Government Printing Office, 1888), 885.

24. *The Medical and Surgical History of the War of the Rebellion*, vol. 1, pt. 3 (Washington, DC: Government Printing Office, 1888), 885.

25. DeWitt C. Peters, "Remarks on the Evils of Youthful Enlistments and Nostalgia," *American Medical Times* (14 Feb. 1863): 75–76.

26. Peters, "Remarks on the Evils," 75.

27. William A. Hammond, M.D., *A Treatise on Insanity in Its Medical Relations* (New York: D. Appleton, 1883; Reprint edition Arno Press, 1973) 411–413.

28. Peters, "Remarks on the Evils," 75.

29. *The Medical and Surgical History of the War of the Rebellion*, vol. 1, pt. 3 (Washington, DC: Government Printing Office, 1888), 886.

30. *The Medical and Surgical History of the War of the Rebellion*, vol. 1, pt. 3 (Washington, DC: Government Printing Office, 1888), 886.

31. *The Medical and Surgical History of the War of the Rebellion*, vol. 1, pt. 3 (Washington, DC: Government Printing Office, 1888), 886.

32. Peters, "Remarks on the Evils," 76.

33. George Worthington Adams, *Doctors in Blue: The Medical History of the Union Army in the Civil War* (Dayton, OH: Press of Morningside, 1985), 137–139.

34. David M. Rein, *S. Weir Mitchell: As a Psychiatric Novelist* (New York: International Universities Press, 1952), 20.

35. Rein, *S. Weir Mitchell,* 35.

36. Rein, *S. Weir Mitchell,* 46.

37. J. M. Da Costa, M.D., "On Irritable Heart: A Clinical Study of a Form of Functional Cardiac Disorder and Its Consequences," *The American Journal of the Medical Sciences,* 121 (Jan. 1871): 17–52.

38. Da Costa, "On Irritable Heart," 21.

39. Da Costa, "On Irritable Heart," 20.

40. Da Costa, "On Irritable Heart," 20.

41. Da Costa, "On Irritable Heart," 40.

42. Da Costa, "On Irritable Heart," 28.

43. Da Costa, "On Irritable Heart," 22.

44. Da Costa, "On Irritable Heart," 29.

45. Albert Deutsch, *The Mentally Ill in America: A History of Their Care and Treatment from Colonial Times,* 2nd ed., rev. and enl. (New York: Columbia University Press, 1949), chapters 2, 3, and 6.

46. Dorothy S. Provine, comp., *Preliminary Inventory of the Records of St. Elizabeth's Hospital* (Washington, DC: National Archives and Records Service, General Services Administration, 1981), 1–2.

47. *RG 418.* Records of St. Elizabeth's Hospital. Petition for Involuntary Hospitalization, Sept. 22, 1865.

48. *RG 418.* Records of St. Elizabeth's Hospital. Annual Report of the Operations of the Government Hospital for the Insane for 1861: 17.

49. *RG 418.* Records of St. Elizabeth's Hospital. Letter to the Secretary of the Interior, from the Navy Department, dated Oct. 5, 1861.

50. *RG 418.* Records of St. Elizabeth's Hospital. Letters between the Secretary of War and the Quartermaster General's Office, dated Feb. 9, 1865, and Feb. 10, 1865.

51. *RG 418.* Records of St. Elizabeth's Hospital. Letters between the

Secretary of War and the Quartermaster General's Office, dated Feb. 9, 1865, and Feb. 10, 1865.

52. *RG 418*. Records of St. Elizabeth's Hospital. Letters between the Secretary of War and the Quartermaster General's Office, dated Feb. 9, 1865, and Feb. 10, 1865.

53. *The Medical and Surgical History of the War of the Rebellion,* vol. 1, pt. 1 (Washington, DC: Government Printing Office, 1870), 719–725.

54. *The Medical and Surgical History of the War of the Rebellion,* vol. 1, pt. 1 (Washington, DC: Government Printing Office, 1870), 719–725.

55. Shelby Foote, *The Civil War: A Narrative—Red River to Appomattox* (New York: Random House, 1974), 391–401.

56. Foote, *The Civil War,* 301.

57. Foote, *The Civil War,* 396.

58. Foote, *The Civil War,* 398.

59. John Laffin, *Americans in Battle* (New York: Crown Publishers, 1973), 253.

60. *RG 418*. Records of St. Elizabeth's Hospital. Ninth Annual Report of the Board of Visitors, and the Twelfth Annual Report of the Superintendent of Construction Government Hospital for the Insane for the Year 1863–1864.

61. *RG 418*. Records of St. Elizabeth's Hospital. Case files of Patients, Case No. 1280 Lucas Hoffman, 1864.

62. *RG 418*. Records of St. Elizabeth's Hospital. Letter from Robert Rellem to the Secretary of the Interior, 1862.

63. *RG 418*. Records of St. Elizabeth's Hospital. Register of Cases, 1859–1867.

64. *RG 418*. Records of St. Elizabeth's Hospital. Ninth Annual Report of the Board of Visitors, and the Twelfth Annual Report of the Superintendent of Construction Government Hospital for the Insane for the Year 1863–1864.

65. *RG 418*. Records of St. Elizabeth's Hospital. Tenth Annual Report of the Board of Visitors, and the Thirteenth Annual

Report of the Superintendent of Construction of the Government Hospital for the Insane, for the Year 1864–1865: 12.

66. *RG 418*. Records of St. Elizabeth's Hospital. Tenth Annual Report of the Board of Visitors, and the Thirteenth Annual Report of the Superintendent of Construction of the Government Hospital for the Insane, for the Year 1864–1865: 10.

67. *RG 418*. Records of St. Elizabeth's Hospital. Tenth Annual Report of the Board of Visitors, and the Thirteenth Annual Report of the Superintendent of Construction of the Government Hospital for the Insane, for the Year 1864–1865: 11.

68. *RG 418*. Records of St. Elizabeth's Hospital. Tenth Annual Report of the Board of Visitors, and the Thirteenth Annual Report of the Superintendent of Construction of the Government Hospital for the Insane, for the Year 1864–1865: 11.

69. *RG 418*. Records of St. Elizabeth's Hospital. Ninth Annual Report of the Board of Visitors, and the Twelfth Annual Report of the Superintendent of Construction Government Hospital for the Insane for the Year 1863–1864: 722.

ENDNOTES TO CHAPTER SEVEN

1. Byron Stinson, "Battle Fatigue and How It was Treated in the CW," *Civil War Times Illustrated*, vol. 4, 7 (Nov. 1965): 43–44.

2. Albert Deutsch, *The Mentally Ill in America: A History of Their Care and Treatment from Colonial Times*, 2nd ed., rev. and enl. (New York: Columbia University Press, 1949), 229–245.

3. James C. Mohr, *Doctors and the Law: Medical Jurisprudence in Nineteenth-Century America* (New York: Oxford University Press, 1993), 160.

4. Eugene Grissom, M.D., LL.D., "True and False Experts," *American Journal of Insanity* (July 1878): 1–36.

5. Grissom, "True and False Experts," 4.

6. Grissom, "True and False Experts," 15.

7. Grissom, "True and False Experts," 18.

8. Grissom, "True and False Experts," 25.

9. Grissom, "True and False Experts," 35.

10. Mohr, *Doctors and the Law*, 177.

11. John P. Gray, "Homicide: Plea, Insanity," *American Journal of Insanity* (Jan. 1865): 388.

12. National Archives. J.A.G. Records LL1431. "Great Jail Outbreak—Escape of Seven Prisoners from Chemung County Jail by Tunneling—Stewart among the Number," *Elmira Daily Gazette*, 25 Jan. 1865.

13. National Archives. J.A.G. Records LL1431. Letter from LeRoy Shear to President Rutherford B. Hayes, 1878

BIBLIOGRAPHY

BOOKS

Adams, George Worthington. *Doctors in Blue: The Medical History of the Union Army in the Civil War.* Dayton, OH: Press of Morningside, 1985.

Bartlett, John. *Familiar Quotations,* sixteenth ed. Boston: Little, Brown and Company, 1992.

Benét, S. V., Bvt. Lieut. Colonel. *A Treatise on Military Law and the Practice of the Courts-Martial.* New York: D. Van Nostrand, 1868.

Billings, John D. *Hardtack and Coffee or the Unwritten Story of Army Life.* Boston: George M. Smith, 1887.

Catton, Bruce. *Bruce Catton's Civil War: Three Volumes in One.* New York: Fairfax Press, 1984.

Davis, George B., Major-General. *A Treatise on the Military Law of the United States: Together with the Practice and Procedure of the Courts-Martial and Other Military Tribunals.* New York: John Wiley and Sons, 1915.

Deutsch, Albert. *The Mentally Ill in America: A History of Their Care and Treatment from Colonial Time.* 2nd ed., rev. and enl. New York: Columbia University Press, 1949.

Foote, Shelby. *The Civil War: A Narrative—Red River to Appomattox.* New York: Random House, 1974.

Greiner, John M., Janet L. Coryell, and James R. Smither, eds., *A Surgeon's Civil War: The Letters and Diary of Daniel M. Holt, M.D.* Kent, OH: Kent State University Press, 1994.

Hammond, William A., M.D. *A Treatise on Insanity in Its Medical Relations.* New York: D. Appleton, 1883; Reprint edition, Arno Press, 1973.

Humphreys, Charles A. *Field, Camp, Hospital and Prison in the Civil War, 1863–1865.* Freeport, NY: Books for Libraries Press, 1971.

Laffin, John. *Americans in Battle.* New York: Crown Publishers, 1973.

Lande, R. Gregory, and David Armitage, eds. *Principles and Practice of Military Forensic Psychiatry.* Springfield, IL: Charles C. Thomas, 1997.

Linderman, Gerald F. *Embattled Courage: The Experience of Combat in the American Civil War,* New York: Free Press, 1987.

Lowry, Thomas P., M.D. *Don't Shoot That Boy!: Abraham Lincoln and Military Justice.* Mason City, IA: Savas Publishing, 1999.

———. *Tarnished Eagles: The Courts-Martial of Fifty Union Colonels and Lieutenant Colonels.* Mechanicsburg, PA: Stackpole Books, 1997.

Lowry, Thomas P., M.D., and Jack D. Walsh, M.D. *Tarnished Scalpels: The Court-Martials of Fifty Union Surgeons.* Mechanicsburg, PA: Stackpole Books, 2000.

Maeder, Thomas. *Crime and Madness: The Origins and Evolutions of the Insanity Defense.* New York: Harper and Row, 1985.

The Medical and Surgical History of the War of the Rebellion, vol. 1, pt. 1. Washington, DC: Government Printing Office, 1870.

The Medical and Surgical History of the War of the Rebellion, Vol. 1, pt. 3. Washington, DC: Government Printing Office, 1888.

Mohr, James C. *Doctors and the Law: Medical Jurisprudence in Nineteenth-Century America.* New York: Oxford University Press, 1993.

Murdock, Eugene. *Patriotism Limited 1862–1865: The Civil War Draft and the Bounty System.* Kent, OH: Kent University Press, 1967.

Provine, Dorothy S., comp. *Preliminary Inventory of the Records of St. Elizabeth's Hospital.* Washington, DC: National Archives and Records Service, General Services Administration, 1981.

Ray, Isaac. *A Treatise on the Medical Jurisprudence of Insanity.* Cambridge, MA: The Belknap Press of Harvard University Press, 1962.

Rein, David M. *S. Weir Mitchell: As a Psychiatric Novelist.* New York: International Universities Press, 1952.

Smith, Page. *Trial by Fire: A People's History of the Civil War and Reconstruction.* New York: McGraw-Hill, 1982.

Stillwell, Leander. *The Story of a Common Soldier of Army Life in the Civil War: 1861–1865.* 2nd ed. Erie, KS: Franklin Hudson, 1920.

Wiley, Bell Irvin. *The Life of Billy Yank: The Common Soldier of the Union.* Indianapolis: Bobbs-Merrill, 1952.

Winthrop, William. *Military Law and Precedents.* Washington, DC: War Department, Office of Adjutant General, 1886.

———. *Military Law and Precedents.* 2nd edition, rev. and enl. Washington, DC: Government Printing Office, 1920.

PERIODICALS

Brock, R. A., ed. *Southern Historical Society Papers,* vol. 21. Richmond, VA: Broad Foot Publishing, 1990.

Castel, Albert, ed. "Malingering: 'Many . . . Diseases Are . . . Feigned.'" *Civil War Times Illustrated,* 21, no. 5 (August 1977): 29.

Da Costa, J. M., M.D. "On Irritable Heart: A Clinical Study of a Form of Functional Cardiac Disorder and Its Consequences." *The American Journal of the Medical Science,* 121 (January 1871): 17–52.

Daniel McNaughton's Case. 10 Clark and Finnelly *Eng. Rep.* 210(8) (1843): 718.

Gray, John P. "The Case of Dr. David M. Wright, for the Murder of Lieutenant Sanborn—Plea, Insanity," *American Journal of Insanity,* 20 (1864): 286.

———. "Case of Lorenzo C. Stewart," *American Journal of Insanity* (January 1865): 18–21.

———. "Homicide: Plea, Insanity," *American Journal of Insanity* (January 1865): 388.

Grissom, Eugene, M.D., LL.D. "True and False Experts," *American Journal of Insanity* (July 1878): 1–36.

Murdock, Eugene C. "Pity the Poor Surgeon." *Civil War History,* vol. 16, no. 1 (March 1970): 26.

Peters, DeWitt C. "Remarks on the Evils of Youthful Enlistments and Nostalgia." *American Medical Times* (14 Feb. 1863): 75–76.

Robertson, James I. "Military Executions." *Civil War Times Illustrated,* vol. 5, no. 2 (1966): 38–39.

Sharp, Arthur G. "Men of Peace." *Civil War Times Illustrated,* vol. 21, no. 4 (June 1982): 30–37.

Spiegal, Allen D., and Florence Kavaler. "Abraham Lincoln, Medical Jurisprudence, and Chloroform—Induced Insanity in an 1857 Murder
Trial." *Caduceus* (Winter 1994): 145–160.

Stinson, Byron. "Battle Fatigue and How It was Treated in the CW." *Civil
War Times Illustrated,* vol. 4, no. 7 (November 1965): 43–44.

Swart, Stanley L. "The Military Examination Board in the Civil War: A Case
Study." *Civil War History,* vol. 16, no. 3 (September 1970): 228.

Wiley, Bell I. "The Common Soldier of the Civil War." *Civil War Times Illustrated,* Special Issue (1973): 48.

NEWSPAPERS

National Archives. J.A.G. Records LL1431. *Elmira Daily Gazette,* 1 Nov.
1863.

National Archives. J.A.G. Records LL1431. "General Count-Martial." *Elmira Daily Gazette,* 2 Dec. 1863.

National Archives. J.A.G. Records LL1431. "The Stewart Desertion and
Murder Case." *Elmira Daily Gazette,* 23 Dec. 1863.

National Archives. J.A.G. Records LL1431. "All Hopes Gone." *Elmira Daily
Gazette,* 21 Apr. 1864.

National Archives. J.A.G. Records LL1431. "Suspension of Stewart's Sentence." *Elmira Daily Gazette,* 24 Apr. 1864.

National Archives. J.A.G. Records LL1431. "Great Jail Outbreak—Escape
of Seven Prisoners from Chemung County Jail by Tunneling—Stewart
among the Number." *Elmira Daily Gazette,* 25 Jan. 1865.

PRIMARY SOURCE DOCUMENTS

General Court-Martial Orders 1, Army of the Potomac, 1865.

General Court-Martial Orders 13, Department of Missouri, 1882.

General Court-Martial Orders 29, Department of Missouri, 1869.

General Court-Martial Orders 35, Army of the Potomac, 1864.

General Court-Martial Orders 39, Department of Missouri, 1868.

General Orders 5, Department of the Pacific, 1864.

General Orders 7, War Department, 1856.

General Orders 10, Department of the Gulf, 1866.

General Orders 12, Army of the Potomac, 1865.

General Orders 13, Northern Department, 1864.

General Orders 22, Department of North Carolina, 1865.

General Orders 25, Department of New Mexico, 1862.

General Orders 30, Department of Missouri, 1864.

General Orders 31, Department of Washington, 1865.

General Orders 33, Department of Ohio, 1863.

General Orders 37, Middle Department, 1864.

General Orders 43, Department of Virginia and North Carolina, 1864.

General Orders 45, Department of the Pacific, 1863.

General Orders 48, Department of Virginia, 1864.

General Orders 53, 98, Army of the Potomac, 1862.

General Orders 54, Department of the Pacific, 1864.

General Orders 74, Department of Washington, 1865.

General Orders 74, Middle Department, 1864.

General Orders 80, Department of Missouri, 1864.

General Orders 91, Army of the Potomac, 1863.

General Orders 96, Department of New Mexico, 1862.

General Orders 101, Department of Missouri, 1864.

General Orders 122, Department of Missouri, 1864.

General Orders 126, Department of Missouri, 1864.

General Orders 132, Department of the Gulf, 1864.

General Orders 153, Department of Missouri, 1864.

General Orders 178, Department of the Gulf, 1864.

National Archives. J.A.G. Records LL1431. E. D. Townsend, Assistant Adjutant General. "To Major General Dix." 21 Apr. 1864. Copy of a Telegram.

National Archives. J.A.G. Records LL1431. Letter from LeRoy Shear to President Rugterford B. Hayes, 1878.

National Archives. J.A.G. Records LL1431. Letter from Private Stewart to President Abraham Lincoln from Chemung County Jail, 30 Mar. 1864.

National Archives. J.A.G. Records LL1431. A letter from Lorenzo C. Stewart while incarcerated in Chemung County Jail, dated 20 April 1864, Elmira, NY.

National Archives. J.A.G. Records LL1431. Letter from President Abraham Lincoln to Dr. John P. Gray, Utica, NY. In the matter of the inquiry into the mental condition of Lorenzo C. Stewart, April 1864.

National Archives. J.A.G. Records LL1431. Transcript of the Special Court of Inquiry, April–May 1864: 18–19.

National Archives. *RG 48*. Department of the Interior. Correspondence between Dr. Duhamel and the Secretary of the Interior, 1867.

National Archives. *RG 48*. Department of the Interior. Jail Record Books, 1865.

National Archives. *RG 48*. Department of the Interior. Letter and Reward Poster from an inspector at the U.S. Jail to the Secretary of the Interior, 1860.

National Archives. *RG 48*. Department of the Interior. Record Book, 1862.

National Archives. *RG 48*. Department of the Interior. Report of the Warden from the U.S. Jail, July 1865.

National Archives. *RG 48*. Department of the Interior. Report of the Warden of the Jail, Nov. 1865.

National Archives. *RG 48*. Department of the Interior. Rules and Regulations, House of Refuge, Baltimore, MD, circa 1865.

National Archives. *RG 48*. Department of the Interior. Rules and Regulations of the United States Jail, 1857.

National Archives. *RG 48*. Department of the Interior. U.S. Jail Docket, 1863.

National Archives. *RG 48*. Department of the Interior. U.S. Jail Docket, 1865.

National Archives. *RG 94*. *Records of the Adjutant General's Office.* Case of Charles Sperry, file no. NN2427, roll no. 7. Also see General Orders 31, Department of Washington, 1865.

National Archives. *RG 94*. *Records of the Adjutant General's Office.* Case of Darius Philbrooks, file no. II953, roll no. 7. Also see General Orders 25, Department of New Mexico, 1862.

National Archives. *RG 94*. *Records of the Adjutant General's Office.* Case of George W. McDonald, file no. LL2430, roll no. 3. Also see General Orders 74, Middle Department, 1864.

National Archives. *RG 94*. *Records of the Adjutant General's Office.* Case of Henry Hamilton, file no. LL2628, roll no. 2. Also see General Orders 132, Department of the Gulf, 1864.

National Archives. *RG 94*. *Records of the Adjutant General's Office.* Case of Henry Holt, file no. MM1427, roll no. 2. Also see General Orders 43, Department of Virginia and North Carolina, 1864.

National Archives. *RG 94*. *Records of the Adjutant General's Office.* Case of James Preble, file no. MM1774, roll no. 7. Also see General Orders 22, Department of North Carolina, 1865.

National Archives. *RG 94. Records of the Adjutant General's Office.* Case of James Weaver, alias N. E. Baker, file no. OO316, roll no. 8. Also see General Orders 12, Army of the Potomac, 1865.

National Archives. *RG 94. Records of the Adjutant General's Office.* Case of Larkin Ray, file no. NN3261, roll no. 7. Also see General Orders 178, Department of the Gulf, 1864.

National Archives. *RG 94. Records of the Adjutant General's Office.* Case of Michael Wert, file no. LL2924, roll no. 8. Also see General Court-Martial Orders 1, Army of the Potomac, 1865.

National Archives. *RG 94. Records of the Adjutant General's Office.* Case of William Lynch, file no. 2533, roll no. 3. Also see General Court-Martial Orders 35, Army of the Potomac, 1864.

National Archives. *RG 94. Records of the Adjutant General's Office.* "List of U.S. Soldiers Executed by United States Military Authorities during the Late War," 1885.

National Archives. *RG 94. Records of the Adjutant General's Office.* M1523, "Proceedings of U.S. Army Courts-Martial and Military Commissions of Union Soldiers Executed by U.S. Military Authorities, 1861–1866."

National Archives. *RG 418.* Records of St. Elizabeth's Hospital. Annual Report of the Operations of the Government Hospital for the Insane for 1861.

National Archives. *RG 418.* Records of St. Elizabeth's Hospital. Case files of Patients, Case No. 1280, Lucas Hoffman, 1864.

National Archives. *RG 418.* Records of St. Elizabeth's Hospital. Letter from Robert Rellem to the Secretary of the Interior, 1862.

National Archives. *RG 418.* Records of St. Elizabeth's Hospital. Letter to the Secretary of the Interior, from the Navy Department, dated Oct. 5, 1861.

National Archives. *RG 418.* Records of St. Elizabeth's Hospital. Letters between the Secretary of War and the Quartermaster General's Office, dated Feb. 9, 1865, and Feb. 10, 1865.

National Archives. *RG 418.* Records of St. Elizabeth's Hospital. Ninth Annual Report of the Board of Visitors, and the Twelfth Annual Report of the Superintendent of Construction Government Hospital for the Insane for the Year 1863–1864.

National Archives. *RG 418.* Records of St. Elizabeth's Hospital. Petition for Involuntary Hospitalization, Sept. 22, 1865.

National Archives. *RG 418*. Records of St. Elizabeth's Hospital. Register of Cases, 1859–1867.

National Archives. *RG 418*. Records of St. Elizabeth's Hospital. Tenth Annual Report of the Board of Visitors, and the Thirteenth Annual Report of the Superintendent of Construction of the Government Hospital for the Insane, for the Year 1864–1865.

INDEX

ABOUT THE AUTHOR

R. GREGORY LANDE, D.O., is a physician and retired Army Colonel. During his military career, Dr. Lande developed the U.S. Military Forensic Psychiatry Program and was a consultant to the Army Surgeon General on such matters. After retiring from military service, Dr. Lande assumed the position as the Deputy and Director of Professional Services at the William S. Hall Psychiatric Institute, a three hundred-bed hospital in Columbia, South Carolina. In addition to his clinical administrative position, Dr. Lande is an active forensic psychiatrist engaged in the fascinating interface between medicine and the law. He was the lead editor of *The Principles and Practice of Military Forensic Psychiatry*, a textbook devoted to this unique subject.